Dedication

I dedicate my book to the many people especially my colleagues in psychiatry and education who have encouraged and supported me. I have to specifically mention and thank profusely Dr Margaret Wright and Dr Kusay Hadi.

None of this book, of course would have been possible without the experiences that my young clients have brought my way. In trusting me they have shown how encouragement can allow their natural creative abilities to heal their hurts.

There are four people who have to be mentioned and thanked in this dedication. Firstly I thank my wife Diane. Without her warm encouragement this book would never have been finished. Secondly thanks to our friend psychologist, author and artist Vibeke Skov who 'demanded' years ago (in a friendly way) that a record should be made of my 'pioneering work'. Practical help came from Sheila Harvey and Rose Mepham. Thanks to them for keeping the narrative moving onward.

Very special thanks have to go to those who unknowingly, have encouraged me to enthusiastically continue my work; my wonderful children and grandchildren. Through their art and conversations they have constantly inspired me and this inspiration helped me on whenever I faltered.

British Library Cataloguing in Publication Data. A catalogue record for this book is available from the library.

ISBN No: 978 090 484 738 3

Design and artwork by Dylan Jeavons (www.dylandesign.co.uk).

Printed in the UK by Regal Litho Limited.

Contents

About Trevor Jeavons

M.A., Dip Art Th., Dip Ed., N.D.D.

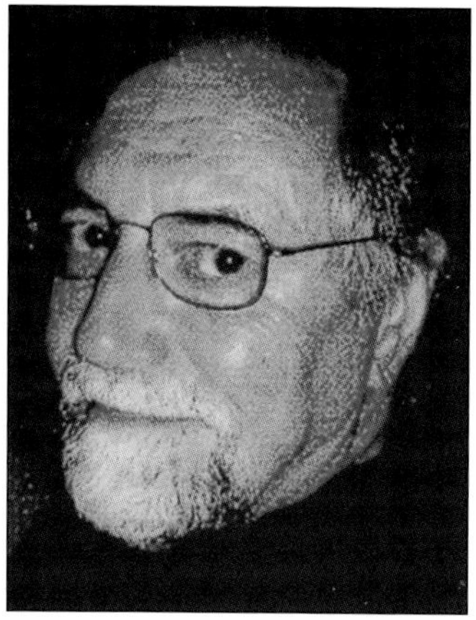

Pioneer therapist, artist and musician. Member of the British Association of Art Therapists.

Trained as a painter, exhibiting mostly in London, alongside such worthies as David Hockney and Mario Dubsky in the 60s. Taught by Bowyer and Palmer (who taught Peter Blake) at Gravesend Art School.

Trevor became increasingly interested in Art as Therapy/Communication, working with severely disabled children, some with brief lives. Studying at London University and University of Hertfordshire. Over the past thirty years he has lectured by invitation in the UK, Iceland, Norway, Switzerland, Portugal, Israel and Denmark. In addition to the UK he is regularly involved in art therapy training programmes in Denmark and Norway.

With Michael Brophy of the Spastics Society, Trevor organised the first exhibition of works by disabled artists at the Royal Academy, London, in 1976.

When Trevor embarked on his teaching career, at first in mainstream and then in special education, he became increasingly interested in the use of art as a therapeutic tool and as an aid to the communication of feelings.

In 1979 Trevor began a new Special School (Oliver Wells), with Nursery, Middle, Senior School, Physiotherapy and Resource Centre in the New City of Milton Keynes for the Buckinghamshire County Council Education Authority. (In 1983 BBC2 TV created a fantasy 'Space Station Milton Keynes'. Partly based on Trevor and the Oliver Wells School).

Because of his innovative work in special education and with the local community, Trevor was one of a number of Milton Keynes professionals invited to lunch with the Queen in 1987. Trevor retired from his role as head teacher in 1990 to concentrate more fully on art therapy and counselling. His first appointment was working with people affected by alcohol and drug abuse, a two year placement in Northampton.

From Northampton, Trevor moved to work for the NHS in Milton Keynes, once more with children. He was until 2006 Senior Art Therapist at the Department of child and Adolescent Psychiatry at the city's hospital, regularly accepting students and mature art therapists from the UK and abroad for training and supervision. Although now retired from that post, he is currently involved on a consultative capacity with the Department. Originally trained as a painter, Trevor exhibited mainly in London at this time and has continued to paint and exhibit his work throughout his career. He is also an accomplished jazz pianist who has performed regularly since 1958. He has found that by maintaining his own creative processes, he has been able to stay more sensitively attuned to those with whom he works

In 'Healing Art and Young People' he shares a wide breadth of personal experience of working in therapy and education with those with special needs.

Now 'partly-retired', Trevor is concentrating on painting, playing and recording jazz piano and still remains involved internationally as a consultant and lecturer in Art Psychotherapy.

Foreword

by Julie Bryant, Art Therapist

This compilation of short case studies by Trevor Jeavons spans many years of his art therapy work with children.

The book includes excerpts from his experiences of working both as an art teacher and also as head of two special schools, even before he began his art therapy training. These examples portray how, even then, he creatively adapted everyday objects and tools to enable creative exploration and mark-making by children with severe physical disabilities.

Recently, Trevor told me how, to his surprise, he was visited in 1972 when he was deputy principal at a residential special school, by a head tutor and founder member and trainees of the then innovative course of art therapy at St Albans. The trainees had come to witness the pioneering work he had instigated with the children – and only then did Trevor realise that he was an art therapist! Many of the challenges of working with this client group are explored within the chapters of Healing Art and Young People. He gives examples of how he and the children involved rose to these challenges, using his innovative ideas to encourage the children's independence, motivation and ability to make choices and their 'mark' upon the world.

To put this in the historical context of approaches towards disability in the 1960s, Trevor's ideas may have been seen as contrary to the often pervading attitudes to the disabled at that time, as being dependent and generally institutionalised.

By the early 1970s, Trevor had already conducted research with the Spastics Society (now Scope). In 1976, he co-ordinated the first exhibition of works by disabled artists at the Royal Academy, London.

It wasn't until the 1980s that Trevor undertook his MA in art therapy, where he continued to contribute his particular knowledge and experience. While on the course he conducted further research into infant drawing and mark-making. The section titled 'Using Art to Improve Communication' includes many of his thoughts and ideas which arose from this period of his career, notably the concept of the 'favoured configuration' – the repeated return to pre-language concepts and mark-making – which was a revolutionary idea.

Trevor elaborates on the importance of pre-representational mark-making, which elevates the scribble or doodle to that which may contain particular personal significance, as well as experimental or explorative value. He warns that markings and drawings from infants should not be viewed in the same light as those made by older people.

Included in the chapter 'Sam's Story of a Journey' are Trevor's reflections on children's reponses to a number of sessions in a mainstream school in 1980. There he invited groups of children to use free undirected drawings on the theme of telling a story of personal significance to them. Sam's story is a moving description which demonstrates how children are often able to use metaphorical equivalents to help express and process their feelings about their life circumstances, if given the opportunity to do so.

The first chapters of this compilation include beautifully described examples from Trevor's work within a multidisciplinary NHS team in an outpatient setting. It is enlightening to find observations from the art therapy trainees' perspective, as well as descriptions of Trevor's approach as the supervisor while working alongside trainees. His writing provides a valuable and perhaps unique insight into two people working together and thinking about the child's developing therapeutic process. His emphasis is on allowing this to unfold and evolve and he highlights the importance of the therapist's ability to bear the ambiguity of not always knowing what is being played out in the child's mind.

Another thought provoking aspect which seems to run like a thread through Trevor's description of his work emphasises the importance of building rapport with the parents and carers of the children in therapy. This has rarely been written about elsewhere.

Trevor's diplomatic, humble and highly sensitive approach has helped to communicate something of his understanding of the child's innermost feelings to those involved in the children's care, which in turn has led to better communication between them and more sustained, positive outcomes in many cases.

On a personal note I would like to add that it is truly a privilege to be acquainted with Trevor. I believe that his warmth, humour and generous nature, combined with his in-depth knowledge and extensive experience in art therapy has inspired not only myself but also many others who have been lucky enough to work with him.

Julie Bryant

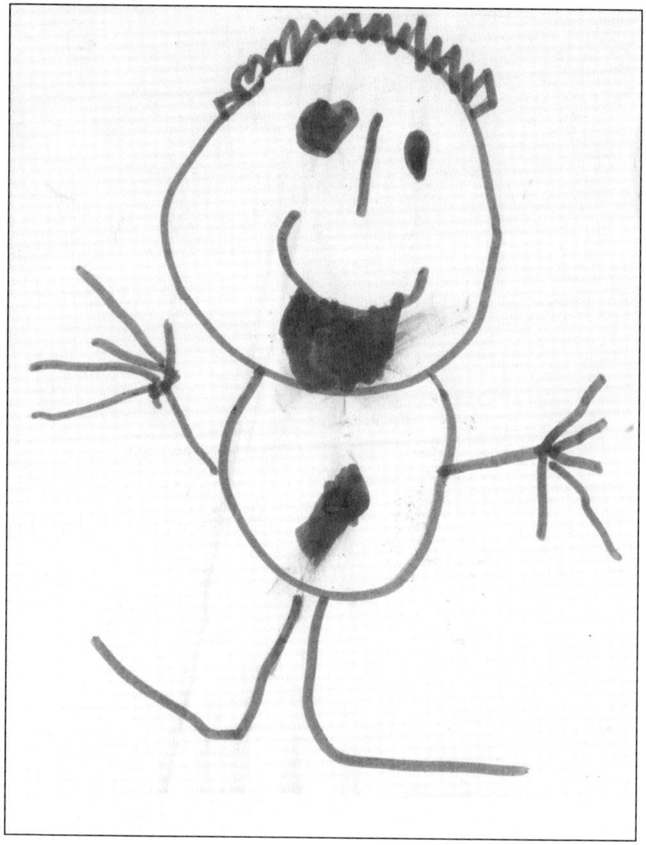

Comments by Vibeke Skov

Clinical Psychologist, artist and author. Director of 'Institute of Art Therapy', Gadbjerg, Denmark and 'School of Art Therapy' Trondheim, Norway.

This book is a wonderful contribution to the field of art therapy. Trevor's long-life experience and understanding of the healing force of symbols and the non-traditional approach to images is truly coming from the heart of an art therapist who knows the world of symbols from the inside.

It seems as if the children can sense his understanding and respect of whatever they bring forward in the therapy room, and therefore can express themselves freely and without the restriction of most adults' rejection of the symbolic reality. The fact is that this approach to development and change works. Children actually get better and their lives improve in quality. And you may wonder what magic was in play. As a Jungian psychologist I am of course fascinated by the many symbols presented by the children. Adam's golden egg would, for instance, be a powerful expression for the true self being activated in the unconscious brought to life simply because the unconscious mind needs that symbol in order to heal itself.

The point being presented in this book is that when first the symbols have been expressed, development can begin its journey towards balance without further interpretation. The starting point is to activate the symbol so that it can begin to work in the psyche and in order to do this, the child needs the freedom to listen to the inside in order to bring that inside out in a creative expression. Together with Trevor in the art therapy room, this is the first magic. I believe that the sharing of the imaginative stories is also a big help for the child in order to accept their importance, so that the healing can come about.

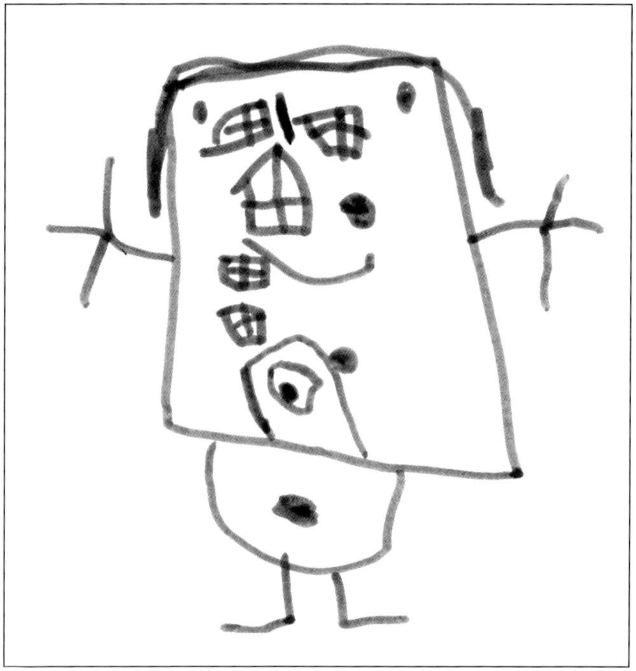

In the book Trevor shares with the reader much of what he has developed during his work with children and I believe that the most important one is the 'listening approach'. A non-judgemental approach to the unconscious seems to be the most effective way to healing.

Trevor has been teaching students in an art therapy training in Denmark, using the same approach as he describes in his book. For more than 20 years I have experienced the effect of his work with adults, and the same magic is happening every time. Students get in touch with their inner symbols and they share their stories with Trevor and each other, and balance is recreated. I often wonder if this sharing of the imaginative reality is what we truly need in our society, as rituals that heal, not only the individual but the outside world as well.

Vibeke Skov

Introduction

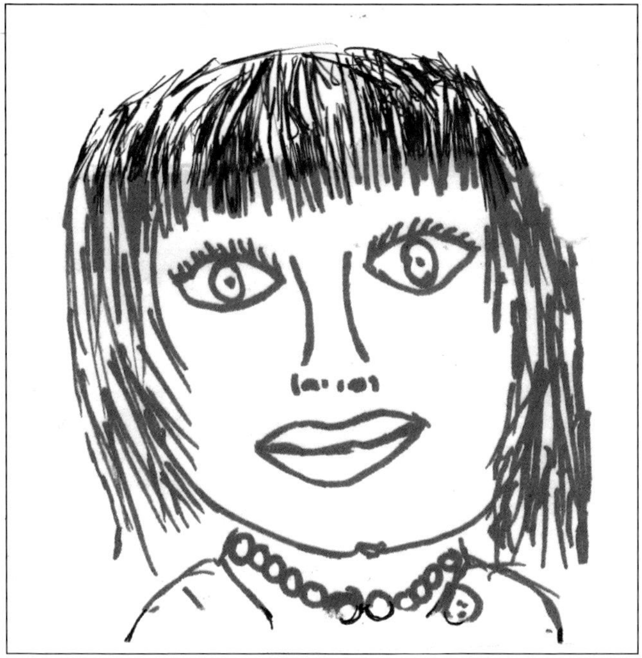

This book tells true stories of young people who are greatly helped, or even healed, by their own artwork. The reader requires no knowledge of psychiatry or medicine, as each chapter tells it just 'how it is'.

The author has worked with emotionally disturbed young people, including those attempting suicide, disadvantaged by disability and even those with very brief lives. The stories here begin with Adam and his clay snowman who delivers great wisdom. Magical and heart-warming, true tales and experiences with fairies, space adventures, dreamscapes and descriptions of the author's journey are presented as easy reading with a minimum of technical comment.

Later chapters refer to work with the physically handicapped and a researched view of infantile artwork.

While all the accounts are accurate, names have been changed to protect the young artists concerned.

Chapter 1

Art Therapy... and Adam

Adam looked older than his six-and-a-half years. His big brown eyes peeped out from under a fringe that needed some attention. "Do you like my snowman?" he asked.
"Very much, I think it's very special," I replied.
The 'snowman' was in fact a lump of unpainted wet clay held between Adam's stubby fingers. There were no details on the figure and it might have been seen as naïve, crude and unfinished. To me, sitting in the little messy art-room surrounded by scores of paintings and models, Adam's snowman was special and unique.
I have seen over the years many snowmen emerge from clay but I have never specifically requested one. 'Do whatever you want' is the rule in my art-room; most children love snowmen and when they make one it is of course important and unique to them and shown off with pride. Of course I like the model; of course it is a wonderful snowman.
"Did you know?" Adam was then very serious and he looked away from me to concentrate on the model he was holding.
"Know what?" I asked.
"Snowmen melt, don't they, Trevor?"
"Always... I suppose."
"Yes they do." Then he paused. The room seemed very still. Adam spoke quietly.
"And they are sad... but the snow-water goes back into the sky... comes back again next winter." His face lit up. "The snowmen know this... but they still feel sad to go."

As happened frequently, I was amazed by the wisdom from the young. Adam's imagination seemed to have allowed him, as he thought about his little model, to conceive a metaphor for life, death and life again.
After our session, I took Adam to the waiting room and sought a few quiet words with his mother. Adam seemed uninterested in my approach to her and busied himself playing with the toys that littered the floor. I knew that Adam's mother had been told that she had cancer and could only expect to live, at the most, another year.
"How was he?" she asked.
I told her of the wonderful snowman story and asked her if she knew where he had found the idea. Interestingly, she insisted that he had no books about snowmen and had never mentioned hearing such a tale at school. She told me later that on the way home she had enquired about 'snowmen' and Adam had replied, "I just made that up for Trevor."

Although I sometimes work with adults, I have specialised in one-to-one psychiatric work with children, mostly in the hospital day clinic. Much of what follows here is about images and stories from the patients and clearly for the patients; the therapist is the facilitator allowing them to help themselves.

I do not profess to work in any one mode of art therapy. I have adopted an eclectic approach, which I suppose is influenced by various psychotherapeutic theories relevant to both projective therapies and counselling. I am also influenced by an understanding of my own creative processes, as well as my previous experiences, including that of head teacher of two 'special schools'. In addition to this, during and before my art therapy training I conducted detailed studies into the mark-making behaviour of infants and children. This latter experience I found especially helpful when working with the under-sixes.

I respect every patient who comes my way. In my view, each has unique abilities and unique disabilities. Whatever the term given to the patient's problem (and a label can sometimes be helpful), that difficulty is in fact a singular problem with different causes and influences. The way that I move through a process of art therapy with patients is defined by their very individual needs. These are perhaps never fully discovered but many become apparent as we work together. The reality is often very different from the file-notes. I firmly believe that the creativity of the art therapist is fundamental to finding a positive and necessarily unique way of working together (i.e. the patient and the therapist). My role is to be 'suspended in a receptive way' beside the client, totally focussed on the therapeutic situation and ready for the most suitable way of working to become apparent to him or to us both.

Strangely, I frequently feel that I am doing very little in some sessions but when my work is video-recorded I see that surprisingly, much is always happening. Movements and gestures and variations in tone of my verbalisation are clearly useful and mostly unconsciously occurring. 'Improvisation' is often the key word.

A trainee student wrote the following some years ago, after working closely with me:

'The therapy begins as soon as he collects the child from the waiting room. His greeting and conversation can all be important foundations for the session to come. He has a basically non-directive approach and explains to the client that it is their time to use as they choose and that the only boundaries are those of time: the length of time, the length of each session and the number of sessions. No themes or structures are imposed and it is emphasised that the client is free to draw to draw and/or talk about what they wish, whenever they want to.

'The art therapist believes that giving the client full choices and opportunities to make decisions can validate his or her feelings, thoughts, opinions, likes or dislikes. This can lead to the child using their own personal resources and improving their own self-confidence. He wants the art room to be a safe space for the client's self-exploration and self-discovery. He uses a variety of techniques to implement this; sometimes he will just "be" with the child and observe their drawing, painting and modelling; often he will draw with the client, on the client's request, or work alongside, working on his own piece of art. This drawing would be relevant to the session, often depicting what he feels is happening, or relating directly to the client. He may choose to share its content with the client or use it for reference for his notes. A drawing he did without prompting during a session while the client was absorbed in their own work depicts a boy stuck up a tree. The art therapist admitted later that he had felt 'stuck' in the session, unsure how to help the client or if, indeed, he could help him. At the end of the session he showed it to the boy, saying that he had done a drawing of how he was feeling and asked if the boy felt like this sometimes. He gave the client an opportunity to transfer the client's own feelings of frustration and despair onto his own drawing, in such a way that he was offering direction but leaving it up to the child whether he took it or not.

'An accepting, non-judgemental and understanding therapeutic relationship provides a foundation for healing and personal growth. It may provide the relatively new experience of feeling valued, safe, held and able to risk expressing and exploring difficulties and anxieties...'

For the 'discovery' of image and narrative to have an effectively therapeutic meaning, it has to emerge from the client him/herself at their own pace. I prefer not to offer interpretations. I would rather the client made their own sense of their work, believing that my interpretation can be limiting. If an image is interpreted, the art therapist can impose his or her ideas, expectations and hopes onto it. It can be taken by the patient to signify the therapist's control or superiority. As the image is tangible and timeless, the art therapist can be accepting of the image and show that he is open to its multiple potential meanings. This gives space and time for the client and therapist to allow understandings to filter through, to allow positive responses to the 'feel' of what is occurring. Whether or not the therapist responds to the symbols that appear or to the comments the patient makes, it is surely that very special overall feeling that guides the therapist's response and makes the journey of healing effective.

I realise that when embarking on art therapy the child is often experiencing profoundly conflicting emotions. The making of the art object can give the child a chance to 'take over', even within a fantasy, an aspect of their life (this is especially important if other circumstances in their life have left them powerless). The patient is able to make sense of things and have some control over them by giving form to feeling. My personal view is that greater powers are witnessed when the patient introduces fanciful descriptions and narratives, which gives extra life to their images. When I ask, "Is there also a story about it?" I am usually told, "Yes," and a story follows for me to scribble down, (There is very much a bias towards the patient's use of narrative in my case choices in this book.)

In art therapy, uncomfortable feelings can be safely confronted, situations and experiences examined in metaphor and if the patient's world is in chaos, he or she might give it order.

As much of what follows in this book is about the 'art' within 'art therapy', I would like to make a few comments concerning absence of image.

Usually the work is one-to-one but the communication between the patient and myself almost inevitably includes a 'third party', the creation or 'image' made by the patient. In my view this is one of the differences between art-therapies and talk-therapies but I do realise, having worked earlier in my career as a counsellor/talk therapist, that the verbal style and body language content between therapist and patient might be seen in a similar way. Those outside of art therapy may not of course realise that the created image is not always present in the therapist-patient relationship. This is usually overlooked in writing about art therapy. It is not there when we begin and, because my approach to art therapy encourages the patient to take the image away with them, we are frequently without image but awaiting an image.

Contrary to some theories, I find that a little chat helps to relax the communication between the patient and myself. The periods without image are, of course, very important. They help to create the environment in which the image is born and a good birth is very helpful. While the image or images, in paint, clay or whatever, are developing, the development in itself is an important part of the therapy. This is the process. Towards its completion – and there may be ongoing modifications – a particular power enters into the therapy.

This image is the product and much has been written about the values of process and product, but behind all of this in the therapy room is the subtle communication, both verbal and non-verbal, between patient and therapist. This, regardless of what is processed or imaged, can make or break the therapeutic process.

Because of the power of the subtle communication behind the creative interaction between art therapist and patient, there may be surprising developments. One such development may be that, despite promising processes and products, the therapy is minimal or entirely absent due to the lack of in-depth communication between patient and therapist. There is failure. On the other hand, and I have seen this on many occasions, despite an apparent vacuum within the 'art relationship' (for instance, no interest in the process, little relevant comment in discussion and apparently irrelevant product) there may be great success because of the 'therapy relationship' where there has been a very helpful breadth of subtle communication between therapist and patient, perhaps without the therapist's knowledge. So it could be that when it looks as if the work seems promising it may not be, and when little seems to be happening there may be great progress! I do believe therefore, that the subtle communication behind the creative/therapeutic action in the therapy room is extremely important.

In this book I try to avoid jargon. I present encounters with the creative power of children. The creative expression when considered brings healing. I am the facilitator only. The child's unique power is rarely tapped but in the safety of art therapy it may emerge and amaze.

It is a great pity that the imagination of the young, their inventiveness and positive creativity is not greatly valued in general and in particular in education.

Before I took Adam as a patient I had met with his mother. This followed on from receiving the referral letter explaining Adam's disturbed behaviour, which had been sent by the family doctor to our team at the Department of Child and Adolescent Psychiatry at the city hospital. As usual the team, in the weekly referral meetings, led by our senior psychiatrist (clinical director) each read out one of the referral letters. The team comprised psychiatrists, psychologists, family therapists, child psychotherapists, psychiatric nurses and art therapist (myself). The team's opinion was that art therapy, with its absence of direct questioning and supposition, should help Adam.

The letter explained that Adam's behaviour had deteriorated over the past three months, with temper tantrums, bed wetting and waking nightmares. We all thought that, even though no one had told Adam of his mother's illness and limited life expectancy, he was sensitive to at least some of what was occurring and was very much stressed and confused by what he was feeling.

We wrote to Adam's mother and met with her. She was a friendly divorcee in her mid-thirties, looking surprisingly healthy. I explained how art therapy might help her son by allowing him to express, from his imagination, whatever he liked. I even said, "He should find relief from off-loading his fears."
Adam's mother listened and said, "I want no-one to tell Adam of my problem. I will not... but he seems to be sensing something... his behaviour is disturbed but he's been told nothing... if only he could get over this 'stressing stuff' and be his old self."
Despite my optimism when I was with Adam's mother, I later felt that despite the support we might give and whatever relief Adam might gain from his expressions, this all seemed a sad and hopeless situation.

At our next session, Adam greeted me enthusiastically and asked me to draw a dinosaur while he took paint and brushes from the table and began to paint a simple tree. Adam hummed a little tune and seemed to be lost in his work. A smudgy grey shape was added beside the spiky tree. I told Adam that I could see that things were happening in his picture. Unthinkingly I asked Adam if the tree could talk (I'm often told that they do).
He looked at me as if to say, "Of course," but instead immediately began his story:
"This is a grey rabbit by the tree. The tree asks the rabbit, 'Why isn't everything like it should be?' but the rabbit says nothing! So... the tree asks the air, 'Why isn't everything like it should be?' Then the air talks to the tree. 'Because we should stop worrying, then everything will be the same.'"

Adam viewed his picture with a satisfied look upon his face. I was thinking that the story must connect with hope. If only things were the same with Mummy. Perhaps, too, asking about 'things' made 'things' more real, which could be very bad. The 'rabbit' part of the situation is silent. The spiky tree wants to know and the invisible wind perhaps points out that day-to-day things could be well but thinking and talking and worrying about 'things' (his mother's illness and death) is upsetting everything.

Next, Adam, apparently no longer concerned with the picture and story, started looking at the little dinosaur I had drawn. He said that he had drawn a dinosaur at school. I asked if school was enjoyable and Adam said, "Kind of." I asked if all was well at home. Adam smiled. "Yes, it's more fun now. Mummy used to go out to work but now she doesn't... she's at home."
We might gather from this that life was better than before for Adam but his free expressions revealed his deep concern. Someone just talking with Adam might suspect that he had no idea of his mother's condition. His tantrums, moods and wet beds indicated otherwise. I wondered too whether Adam had asked his mother why she was at home rather than at work.

In later sessions Adam talked a great deal. Most of what he had to say was apparently of little consequence but I felt that, given that there were few males in Adam's life, he was making a rather special bond with me. One session was particularly interesting, because instead of inventing a special story or making a special image, Adam chatted while messing about with clay with no image resulting, then after washing his hands wrote his name over and over on paper with coloured pencils. I have found the repeating name to be an act of affirmation, the child affirming his existence and individuality. The session with mud play and name writing may have been a very special therapy for Adam but in such a situation, little is provable.

There was one more session planned for Adam, followed by a review of Adam's progress with his mother. It was likely that we would plan more art therapy even though this was his sixth three-quarter hour session.

Adam came smiling and enthusiastically into the art room with what he said was a great idea. "I'm going to make a clay snake!" We took some clay from the bin and he took nearly half-an-hour carefully perfecting rolling clay into a long snake. He seemed completely lost in his creativity but then, with his eyes still upon his work, he told me that a grass snake had been found by girls at his school but it was dead. As the clay snake was finished Adam told me enthusiastically, "This is the snake when it was alive." There seemed to be lots of thinking going on as the boy made his snake, almost bringing life into it. He was so emphatic that he had made a live snake. So much about hanging on to life and so much about the difference between death and life was, I am sure, being enacted by Adam.

As Adam painted his snake, he talked, for some reason, about fairies. "Fairies?! Some people say they are true... some people say they are not true... but there seems to be Tooth Fairies..."

Then with messy green fingers he took some paper and a pencil from the table and drew a medium-sized fairy with butterfly wings and beside it a similar but tiny fairy. I thought of mother and son but said nothing. Adam put his pencil down, looked and me and frowned. "Are they true, Trevor?"
I was surprised and almost panicked but heard myself say, "What is true?" emphasising the word 'true'. Luckily wise Adam helped. Very thoughtfully he frowned and advised me, "Well, you have to get your own idea. You have to try to see. Look closely and think." That was it! I thanked him.

Sometimes within these sessions, Adam made me feel that he was my therapist. However, it was clear that he found freedom in the art therapy environment; freedom to discover truths and possibilities. He had the power to help himself.

There were to be three more of Adam's special stories before we parted company. His mother was telling me that he was sleeping better, no nightmares or wet beds but he was still easily angered by her and in school. Adam made a 'muddle' of clay, which he said was a group of chickens:
"These chickens got laid by the mum
They ran away from their mum
They went to a far-off land…
There were magic chickens in that land
And these chickens became magic

"They laid golden eggs… and every day!"

"Only one man and a pet dog
Looked after all these chickens
The man took the golden eggs, sold them in another land.
But some he kept for treasure.
Every day this happened."

"The mummy chicken was looking for her chickens in the night.
She looked in a hole… a fox.
Was just waking up and it ate her!
…But at least the children got to live in a far-off land.
"Cos we children have to go out into the world and explore!"

Adam was happy that I was noting his story. "Well done, Adam." I said. It all seemed very symbolic, although much was a mystery to me. I could perhaps guess about the man's golden eggs and be confident about what the Mummy chicken's death is about but what really matters here is what the story's creation does for Adam. Here is a Mummy dying while life continues for her children ('we children'). Later, when Adam's mother heard the story, she was clearly moved.

To my surprise, Adam put his clay back in the bin. "Now you, Trevor," he said. "Make me a little clay man and a little clay lady." I did my best with two very simple little figures not much longer than my first finger. Before I was finished he pushed my pencil towards my paper and launched into the second narrative of the day:
"A man and a woman…
They are normal people
But sometimes they smile.
And one day they
Wanted to split up
And later they met up to talk
About their adventures."

In these stories, I felt, we had optimisms within life's harsh realities; children growing away from parents, divorces and friendships.

In the final session, Adam's mother asked to see me alone before we began. I saw lines of distress in her face and felt for her. But the news was a relief; her cancer had been mis-diagnosed. She was very angry with the specialist but at the same time so relieved. We agreed that this session should be the last. I will never know how much Adam's mother shared with him.

Adam and I had previously talked about 'ending' and after seeing his mother, I explained to him how we could have a relaxed and friendly hour before we said farewell.

Adam seemed very relaxed and busied himself by taking up paper and paints and gently puddled little areas of brown, red and blue. Then he told his tale with little periods of silence but no concerns. I wrote as he spoke:

"A squirrel lived… on a skinny tree. Next to this tree was a bad tree that granted bad wishes! They were deep in the forest. The boy went – and the tree granted a wish – but there was a trick:
If the wish was good – it was bad!
If the wish was bad – it was good!"

(I remembered Adam's tree that asks questions from our first session. This tree seemed more powerful.)

"He had wanted a good wish, so it turned into a bad wish. He ran away. The tree gave him a whirlwind instead of the load of gold the boy wanted! So the boy ran away home."

Here Adam hesitated. It seemed to me that he was thinking of his own home.

"He went back one day with an axe. He saw that the tree was getting old. He saw the squirrel who said, 'Don't trust the tree… he just changed himself with magic,' and the boy said, 'I've got an axe in my hand. I'm going to chop the tree down.'
"The squirrel said, 'You can't… that tree is good for the whole wood… even though it is bad for wishing, because if you chop it down, the wood would be flooded and the flood might go to your house. The only way we can stop it is to go in for a bad wish which will become a good wish… can kill the tree!'

"So the boy made a bad wish – he asked for a skeleton and instead he got lots of gold. Then the tree fell down and died. (No floods came because you have to chop the tree down to make that happen.)"

At the end of this last session when we said goodbye, I was so happy that Adam and his mother would be well. Adam I am sure benefitted from the stories. I certainly benefitted from them and I hope his mother did too. In general I would say that his narrative process from within himself was preparing him for his mother's death. I can never forget the tale of the snowman; I tell it to almost everyone I talk with!
As for 'Once upon a forest?' It is a myth. Perhaps it is about managing the trials and tribulations of life? It seems to originate from very deep within the little boy. In the first session we had a tree and in our last session we had a tree. Somehow to analyse this last tale (if one could!) would rob it of its magic.

I will leave it, like all of Adam's tales, for you to think about! I came across Adam and his mother eighteen months later and both were doing very well.

Looking back on Adam's case, I realise how common it is in my experience for mothers to be surprised that their children have knowledge which has not been relayed to them. Mothers seem almost to forget that their children started life as part of them and they begin communicating with each other long before spoken language begins. Little children are excellent at picking up feelings, especially from their mothers, as communication begins without words, with body and facial movements, gestures and tone of voice.

Adam's unspoken anxieties no doubt connected with all these pre-verbal clues and the seriousness of it all was confirmed by his mother giving up her occupation. Luckily, art therapy gave him the opportunity to find some sense in complex happenings. I felt by the end of each session he had, in a most natural way, offloaded much of his anxiety. He seemed relieved. Happily there was a positive outcome in this case.

Chapter 2

Josephine's Fairies

Like Adam, ten-year-old Josephine felt that she was losing her mother. She was not, however, losing her mother through death but losing the love of her mother through her parent's severe depression.

In the session described in this chapter I was joined by Esther Nielsen, a bright friendly young woman and visiting trainee art therapist from psychologist Vibeke Skov's Institute of Art Therapy in Denmark. Vibeke is an old friend of mine, a pioneer in art therapy who has trained many art therapists in Denmark and Norway. I have worked with her for a number of years and accepted her students for periods of training. While I hope they have gained something from my training, I have certainly learnt much from them and from Vibeke.

Josephine's case is, I believe, a good example of a child in art therapy finding metaphors in fantasy to help her to manage a difficult environment which cannot be, or is unlikely to be, improved. Here the child is supported, not cured. At the time these notes were written, the little girl was still producing images and enactments which made sense of her imaginative world and, I'm sure, assisting her in the real one. This clearly helped her to manage the great difficulty in her life.

The problem was that her mother was not able to feel love or to show love to her. Because of abuse suffered in her infancy, the mother had a very poor image of herself. The more her daughter grew, the more Josephine's mother saw of herself in her and the more the depressive aspects of her illness surfaced. She could not bear even to touch her child. Logically the girl had some comprehension of the situation which had been explained to her but, emotionally, there was little understanding and great pain from this rejection.

The account that follows is taken from notes made by Esther and myself at the time. All ideas were from Josephine but it is the role of the therapist to make things possible and allow the enactment to develop.

'Little Jo leaves the art therapy sessions much relieved and relaxed as her free imaginings make sense of the current state of family dynamics. Because of the mother's continuing depression, art therapy cannot provide a complete cure in this case but, according to the family, provides much support. Jo's themes are usually about building homes, taking them apart and trying again. Sometimes the homes are populated with young girls, or even angry lions. With the surprising appearance of the fairies described here, especially with a mother "stuck" in the cold mud, a wider expression of family dynamics becomes possible in metaphor.

'It is Jo's eighth art therapy appointment with Trevor. She has done a number of exciting drawings and models. We asked and she accepts Esther staying in the room together with us.

'She starts talking to Trevor about her things in her locker in the room and then asks Esther if she wants to see them. Esther can look but Jo says that her things should not come out and that her clay flower is anyway glued to the back of the locker and "should stay there for ever". (Interestingly, Jo never takes her work home.) She has pieces of flat clay which she says can be

"fixed". Today she wants to glue these sides for a birdhouse that she began in an earlier session. We do that all together, taking some time. Jo also shows Esther a little clay bowl in her locker. She explains it is about Trevor; it has a rainbow painted on it and a grey area by the rainbow. Jo laughs and says, "It's all a picture of Trevor!" (Trevor, who has a grey beard, knows about this and joins in with the laughter.) A container is Trevor!

'Trevor asks Jo what she's going to do next and quickly she decides on more clay work, now seemingly uninterested in her birdhouse. While Trevor gets the clay, she starts to make rhythms with her hands drumming on the table – quite good. She goes on making dance rhythms, standing up then with all her body swaying. Esther and Trevor join in with the fun. We are all laughing.

'We sit down and Jo is clapping on the big lump of clay that she now has from Trevor. Then she hits it hard with her fist and Trevor does it as well but not so hard. At one point they build up the clay into a mound but even then Jo does not want to stop the hard work of smashing the clay and flattening it. Jo clearly enjoys using up her energy and although it seems fun, Jo seems to be expressing some anger.

'Eventually she stops and detaches a piece of clay and says to Esther, "Catch!" which Esther does the first time but does not succeed the next and gets a lump of clay on her glasses. Lots of laughs, no bad feelings (although there was an element, we thought, of aggression). Now one piece of clay becomes a mountain and another a volcano, according to Jo.

'She continues playing with the clay and talks about life generally. Suddenly she says, "Shhhhhh! There is a fairy, she's under the table. Be quiet or they're all going to die!" We are very quiet and Jo is bending down and talks to the fairy. Then Trevor says something and she hushes (says 'Shhhh'). Jo says urgently, "Quickly Trevor, make fairy wings!" Trevor quickly takes a piece of paper and makes fairy shapes.

'Jo directs: "There are two… mother and two children…" Jo is very anxious to get the wings, so Esther says, "You must hurry," and then Jo says, "Yes hurry, the mother is dying, because she has lost her wings."

'Jo pushes some of the paper pieces into the little mountain of clay (the mountain mound and the volcano came from the earlier almost violent play, possibly an angry symbol which may have inspired the fairy story) and says that the fairy mum is "stuck and dying" in the grey clay mountain. She gets the wings from Trevor and then we have to close our eyes. All is so very quiet and very serious but Jo is in charge. When she tells us to open our eyes we see that the paper fairy is out of the clay and on the table with the other "models".

'Jo proclaims that the mother (who is still dying) is pregnant but is going to have to feed the baby. Trevor has watery eyes because he is genuinely getting very sad. Jo is now staring at his face, observing his reaction. She says, "You look very sad, why?" Trevor says, "It is such a very, very sad story!" Jo seems satisfied with this and continues.
'She looks so very serious, with her big bright eyes constantly moving from the clay-soiled pieces of paper to our faces, seemingly making sure that we are attentive. Very emotional.

'"We can save the baby but we do need to make an operation!" She gets the mother fairy to a space on the table. At once the room is changed into an operating room, where Jo is the doctor; she's directing and giving orders to us. Trevor distributes "surgeon's masks" (paper towels). The mother fairy is lying in front of Jo on the table. Jo sees that we are sitting comfortably beside her and asks us for "scalpels" (modelling tools) and "operating knife" (scissors). Thus we assist, complete with paper towel masks (held between our

teeth). In between orders, Trevor is drawing a tiny baby fairy on a scrap of paper. Next: "operating knife again!" She is passed the scissors and carefully cuts into the mum-fairy.

'Jo is slowly "taking the baby out". She is also, she says, mending a hole in the mum-fairy's wing. With Trevor's help, the baby fairy is very carefully placed beside the mum.

'After the operation, all fairies are brought to Jo's locker. We still have to be quiet but after the locker is closed we may talk again. Jo leads us in talk about how the mother will feel about the baby: "Will she be well enough to care for it?" she says.

'As we talk about the operation, Jo says that Trevor now has to look after them and remember to give them their medicine every day. She suspects that the "medicine" (she pours a little water in a dish) will be gone when she comes back next time. Jo wants Esther to remind Trevor that he is looking after the fairies and giving them their medicine. She also wants Esther to write a letter to her saying that Trevor did look after the fairies and put the letter in her locker the Friday before Esther finishes her placement at the clinic and returns to her art therapy training in Denmark.

'When Jo returned two weeks later, she checked that Esther had flown safely off to Denmark and talked through the "operation" with Trevor and was concerned that all was well. She looked into her locker and said that the fairies were making good progress and took a letter, "To Jo from Esther", from the back of her locker. The note reassured Jo that Trevor had remembered to care for the family. Next, to some extent she changed her mind, saying that all the fairies needed more treatment. Jo took all the scraps out, placed them on the table and mixed up some water with clay, brushing it lightly upon them all. This family needs a lot of help.

'Apparently no fairies had died but they needed more medicine. Jo said that she was particularly worried about the mother, "because she had been stuck in the cold mud".

Jo took her time and placed everything carefully back in the locker at the end of the session.

'The next time Jo attended art therapy she played with the paper pieces and began to paint a paper box to hold them, which she assured me would be much better than the locker. At one point she explained that problems earlier in the mother fairy's life "made it difficult for her to look after the baby". It was wonderful to see how, without Jo, Esther or myself ever referring to her mother's difficulties, the fairy family appeared to help this little girl to bring her internal world into better order; to bring some self-confidence from her imagination to help her, in part, to understand her mother's lack of love towards her.'

This and other sessions throughout twelve months were clearly positive for Josephine, the fairy episode being the most dramatic. I am sure, as were her parents, that art therapy gave her understanding and strength. As with Adam, it was as if something deep within the child surfaced to help and it was made possible by the environment of freedom and trust that was created by the two therapists.

After a year Jo finished with art therapy, spending much of her time successfully involving herself greatly with the many activities during and after hours that her secondary school offered. I saw her out shopping a year or so later; she looked well.

I learned that Jo's mother attended much-needed therapy herself. I hoped that matters improved for all the family.

Chapter 3

Anxiety Denied but Expressed

The two separate 'free' drawings here were made by an emotionally disturbed eleven-year-old boy. At the time he created them his father was due to go into hospital for a heart operation. The boy's mother had died in hospital four years previously.

The boy's anxiety was manifesting itself by him getting into trouble at school, not through antisocial or inappropriate behaviour but through him forgetting what to do, losing items and (perhaps intentionally) ruining his work. His father reported that the boy was restless at night in bed.

When talking to the psychiatrist, the boy said that he was not at all worried by 'anything'. He said that his life was "fine – no problems." According to him, there was nothing he needed to discuss with the psychiatrist.

He was referred to me for art therapy, as something was clearly wrong, even though the boy denied this. He drew freely and a 'strong robot' appeared. "It has," the boy explained, "been hit in the chest by a missile."

In later sessions, he created a number of cars which featured 'strong engines'. Without being prompted, he added comments regarding and questioning the recuperative power of the 'powerful robot' and the longevity of the cars' engines.

I made no comments about the boy's father's heart condition, although the pictures clearly referred to it, but joined in instead with the boy's descriptions and discussions.

He had found his own way of translating his unspoken and unacknowledged fears into images he could deal with. This way he could begin to work through what was troubling him at his own pace in metaphor rather than in a directly confrontational way.

There was a positive outcome for the boy; all his negative behaviour disappeared.

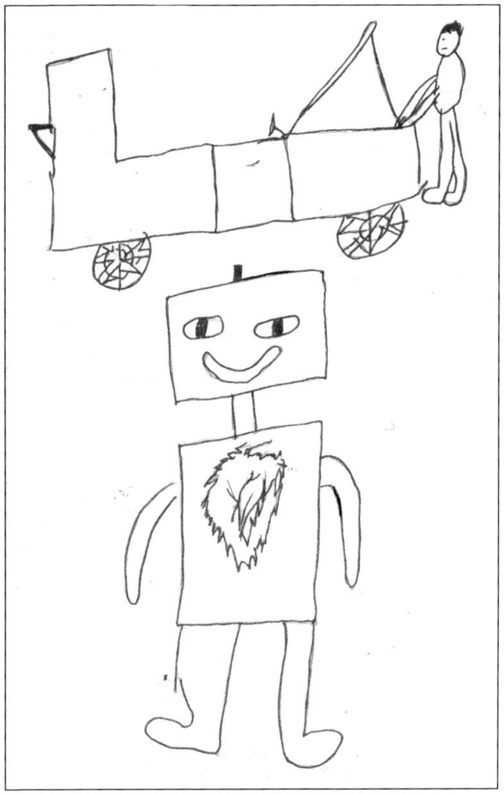

Broken car and damaged robot

Chapter 4

Freddy's Disturbance

Small and usually quiet, Freddy at seven years was an upset boy. His behaviour at school had gone from bad to worse and he was usually a very difficult and moody child at home. The reason for his behaviour was unknown but there was a theory that he was jealous of his baby sister. His mother was a nice and sensible woman who had taken the advice given to her to counteract Freddy's supposed jealousy, but no progress had been made. Freddy's father had been quite unwell for some months and was awaiting a hospital appointment for surgery. I thought that concerns about his father might be contributing to the boy's anxieties.

When I was introduced to Freddy by our senior psychiatrist Dr Margaret Wright, his angry outbursts were continuing and he had recently smashed a number of his favourite toys in a temper tantrum. At the time, Bodil Krezen, another trainee art therapist from Vibeke Skov's course in Denmark, was on a six-week clinical placement under my supervision. I planned to make a beginning with Freddy (a form of assessment for art therapy) with Bodil working beside me, then let her take over from me. She would continue without me being present but I would still meet with her to discuss any developments. My experience with Freddy was very mysterious, as it gave no indication of jealousy.

Given free choice over activity, enthusiastic and friendly Freddy chose to play with clay. He made a simple, stocky little figure about as big as his hand. Freddy clearly liked being in the art-room and talked about the paintings and models, although not about his own little figure.

As he talked, Freddy's clay model developed; unusually exaggerated breasts appeared and lines suggesting clothing. He still made no comment about what it might represent. Bodil and I made a little trivial discussion but interestingly, each of us thought it proper only to congratulate Freddy on his cleverness on making the figure, avoiding questions about what or who it might represent. The appointment came to an end and we arranged to meet the next week, when Freddy intended to paint the model.

At the next session Freddy seemed extremely happy and polite, still delighted with the freedom of our messy art-room. In the waiting room, however, his mother mentioned how much trouble he had been in throughout the past week. Freddy took up the little figure and the poster paints that we had made ready for him. He chose pink and yellow, which he roughly daubed over the surface of the clay. Again, as he worked on the figure, he talked about a number of things to Bodil and myself but not about his creation. Bodil mentioned school and Freddy was happy to relate some of the problems that he had had with a number of children over the past week.

In the middle of all this he commented about his figure: "I need bright orange and red for her booby [breast]." Freddy proceeded to add strong orange and reds to the watery pink and yellow-coloured model, which he said was "the fire of the booby". Freddy's concentration, as he finished the work and took a fresh piece of paper onto the table and carefully placed the figure to one side, seemed to require silence. Bodil and I were very quiet as he drew lines with a pencil. "Just

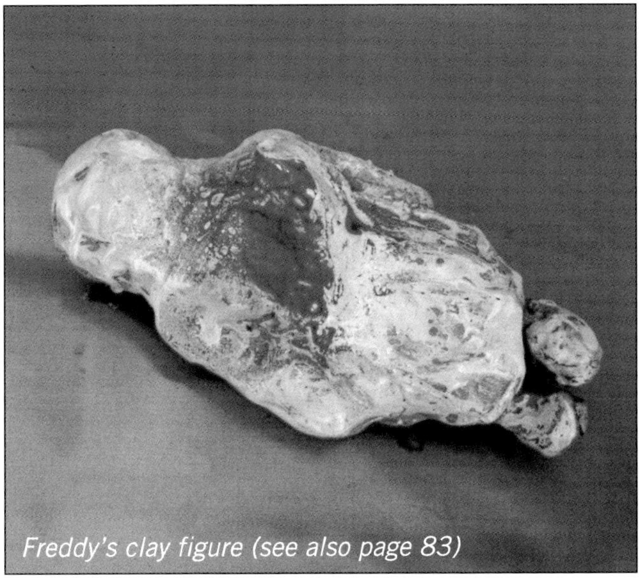

Freddy's clay figure (see also page 83)

lines," Freddy said. There were undulating lines – nothing else – upon the paper but we felt they were meaningful to Freddy. He stood back and looked at the lines with pride.

Realising we were out of time, we allowed Freddy to roll up his drawing and take it to his mother in the waiting room. He seemed to have forgotten his painted model. It was still wet, so when Freddy was gone I placed it carefully in the cupboard and expected Freddy to ask Bodil for it at the next session. Interestingly he did not, referring to it only at his final session. Bodil, sensibly, chose not to bring it out without being asked. She realised that Freddy might have moved on from whatever feeling or idea it represented when he created it.

The third art therapy session was the hand-over to Bodil, the first session where I was not present. Bodil reported:

'Freddy acted a little childishly on this first session with me but seemed happy. He wanted to work with clay and made a spaceship, which turned out to be a crocodile biting someone's back. He crashed it all together, made holes in it and cut it with a modelling stick. This I'm sure represented anger. He decided next that he wanted to paint. He put the clay back into the bucket.

'Next, Freddy got paper, water and paint and he tried to copy a spaceship picture hanging on the wall. After his second try the spaceship became an aeroplane with one deformed wing, which he painted black. The windows he wanted to be white, but the plane became more and more grey. It was "spitting a lot of orange and yellow fire". Black thunder clouds, lightning, blue rain and a helicopter with two propellers appeared next. The sun was hidden behind a big black cloud and Freddy said it would stay there for a little while. The sun "just could not" emerge from behind a cloud, even though Freddy said it might come out. He made no attempt to change the picture. "The sun stays there! He just can't do that!" Three green tree tops are just visible at the bottom of the painting and he said that they look very nice.

'Freddy was very pleased with the stormy picture and said that we should give it to Trevor. At the end Freddy said that he'd really look forward to seeing me next week.'

Bodil and I talked this through. It was clear that Freddy's work was expressing unhappiness. The aircraft was damaged and the storm was angry. Even though Freddy wanted the picture to be brightened up with more colour, to be happier, he had said that he could just not do that. We could not see the crocodile as much else other than a symbol of anger, like the storm.

At the next session Freddy seemed surprisingly happy and content. He came into the room declaring that he wanted to mix lots of colours. Bodil noted:

'Freddy made shades of blues mixed with purples. Shapes... then lines. Despite his happy manner Freddy looked quite serious. The lines were like lines he had

made previously. Freddy commented: "Just scribbles!" Then Freddy grew talkative and told me that his grandmother was visiting this week and that they had been to London all day Tuesday. She will also stay on for Daddy's birthday, he added. I asked him how he had felt over the previous week and he replied that everything had been just fine. It was time to finish and Freddy left very happily, saying, "See you soon!"'

In the next session a week later, his third with Bodil, Freddy was very animated and imaginative. Bodil wrote:

'Freddy said that he wanted to mix colours again, which he did. I had an idea that this time I might join in with the painting. Mine developed as a collection of coloured shapes but Freddy's colours were dark and muddy; browns and dark greys with some black. As soon as Freddy had finished, before I did, he took more paper and some coloured pencils and became extremely busy. He drew the interior of a living room. There is, clearly, a rocking-horse, a television and a window with curtains at the side and lines showing the sun shining through. Through the window the sky which he scribbled blue into. No clouds.

'Freddy moved the picture to one side and took more paper. This time he painted (lots of energy today!) It was a wide rainbow with what he said was a cave under the bow of the rainbow. "You can go in the cave but it's dark inside," Freddy said. Amusingly he told me, "You might find a sleeping bear inside, if you're unlucky. If you're lucky, you could find treasure there, left by pirates." The idea of pirates seemed to excite Freddy and he told me that the pirates would have to make a map so that they could find the treasure again.

'More paper for Freddy; pencils again. He told me that he would draw his grandmother, which he did very well with her sitting in a rocking-chair. Next to grandmother appeared a baby on a rocking-horse with a speech bubble drawn from its mouth saying. "Gaga,gaga." Freddy seemed to join in with the drawn baby by talking in a baby manner as if I were not there; "Mama" noises and "Gaga". Next, grandmother had a speech bubble added which said, "Stop that, baby." Freddy informed me that the baby is six months old and that it might be a girl and it might be a boy. Although I did not say so, it seemed to me that the baby was a very young Freddy.

'In the last minutes of the session Freddy surprised me by remembering his clay figure, which was still in his locker, and asked for it, because he wanted to give it to his mother (which he did on his way out). Freddy's mother received the figure thankfully and happily saying how good it was but, at least at that point, not asking about what it represented.

The session ended with feelings of mystery, especially the presentation of the little clay figure from Freddy to his mother.' The grandmother and baby were intriguing but Bodil and I could not understand what Freddy was expressing. We had both noticed that even though we thought that Freddy's upset was connected with his father's illness, he had never mentioned it.

A week later Bodil and Freddy met again. She notes:

'Freddy's mother told me that it had been a bad week. He had kicked the child-minder (and later had apologised to her) and had been very difficult in school. His mother asked whether he had been in a bad mood because he feared his anti-measles injection and Freddy said that it was the reason.

'During my session he was well-behaved and happy. I asked whether what he had said to his mother was true, or if something else was hidden underneath his angers. Freddy replied that it "really was" about the injection that he was due to have. I did not get round to talking about what mummy thought about the model that he had given her last week.

'Next we did, at Freddy's suggestion, a few fold-together paintings, putting lots of paint on the paper and folding it over. This was quite hurried and because Freddy had said that he wanted to get back to his drawing from our last session (grandmother and baby), we did not get to discuss his colourful patterns.

'I placed the drawing on the table before him and he looked carefully at it and began to make careful decorative scribble on the floor of the room that he had drawn. For some reason I asked Freddy if he had had any interesting dreams lately (perhaps the dream-like quality of his picture caused me to ask). "Yes," he replied, "yesterday." Freddy said that he had not told anyone else about the dream. It was about his picture of a cave under the rainbow:
'Freddy walked up to the cave and peered into the darkness. He could see nothing but felt very brave and thought that there might be treasure in there. When he had crept deep inside suddenly a four-headed dragon rushed up to him, spitting out great flames. But Freddy was, he said, ready for the dragon; he was carrying a shield and he held it up to defend himself.

'Amazingly all the fire was deflected back to the dragon, which was quickly destroyed. There beside the dragon was a pile of treasure (I remembered that dragons liked to collect treasures and guarded them jealously). Freddy picked up gold, silver, diamonds and sparkling jewellery "but it was only a dream".

'At that point Freddy completed the pencilled shading on the bottom of his drawing and it seemed that it was now finished. We had gone over our time together and shared pleasant goodbyes and best wishes to each other. Because of my return to Denmark I would not see Freddy again but he knew this would be our last session. I took Freddy to his mother and it was a nice, friendly ending. His mother thanked me for my help. I explained that Trevor would see her in two weeks' time.'

Before her return to Denmark, Bodil and I discussed in full Freddy's case and we looked back over the sessions: In the first two sessions Freddy produced, from free choice, his detailed painted clay model of a feminine figure with a 'breast of fire' emerging from her blouse. This he eventually gave to his mother. I believe that this was the beginning (with no pre-amble!) of a process of expression and sharing , bordering sometimes on ritual. In this Freddy surely has gained much by putting his expressions from fantasy into some order and through both expressing and through sharing had gained confidence. It seemed important that his mother was given the figure and Trevor the storm painting.

With all of Bodil's information, I arranged to meet with Freddy's mother. We talked about the burning breast and she surprised me as she confided that her breast had been damaged by severe burning she had received in a road accident but that she had persevered with breast feeding with both her children. It is likely that Freddy had noticed this when the baby was being suckled and just possible that he retains infantile memories from his own feeding. There is, I am sure, an echo of this perception of damage in the deformed wing on his painted aircraft.

Freddy had moved on with ease to even deeper expressions over the weeks in therapy with Bodil Krenzen. Her excellent work enabled further interior and exterior communication for Freddy. By this I mean Freddy gained from communication from his inner self to his conscious self and gained also from the relief of sharing with another.

It is enough that Freddy became stabilised emotionally because of these sessions but through his imaginings in art therapy, one can see a development where he is less anxious after bringing his concerns out into the open.

Bodil and I had seen in Freddy's expressions:

1. Anger: e.g. the back-biting crocodile which is destroyed and perhaps especially the stormy paintings.

2. Immaturity: the scene with baby talk – a wish to regress.

3. Security: the living room, the rainbow paintings, the cave.

4. The unspoken concern: the damaged breast (perhaps even guilt if he thinks the feeding child is damaging the breast).

5. Development of confidence: the 'dream' of under the rainbow where much is gained when the monster is bravely conquered. The flames are significant.

These are the more clearly expressed portions of his therapy but the most helpful parts for Freddy (who was emotionally disturbed and confused) may have been those which were most unclear to the two of us, the encouragers and observers.

At our meeting with Freddy's mother, she said that he seemed so much more settled after his art therapy sessions and that his good mood and improved behaviour had so far continued. Real progress.

We had finished our work. Two months later I heard that Freddy's father was in good health after successful surgery. In the New Year, Freddy's parents sent a note of thanks to the clinic and reported that all was fine and that as well as being happier, 'Freddy is so much more grown up these days'.

I cannot be sure exactly what Freddy's art therapy sessions meant but I am sure that he gained relief from expressing his anxieties in a symbolic way. It appeared to be a very positive outcome: by sharing in metaphor through the freedom of art, Freddy seemed to have diminished or lost his fears and returned to a happy state of mind.

Chapter 5

Angry Kenny

The full story of Kenny's process in art therapy would fill a book by itself. I have chosen to detail the final session here, as it involves Kenny's mother and their relationship as they tried to cope with the loss of a husband and father. Kenny's healing was complicated by his mother's bereaved state of mind, which was one of both sadness and anger.

Kenny was a likeable twelve-year-old who was referred to the clinic because of increasingly disruptive behaviour at home and at school. His father, to whom he had been very close, had died nine months previously and the consultant child and adolescent psychiatrist felt that art therapy could help him to work through his bereavement problems. At the same time, his mother was receiving psychiatric help.

This was to be our final session. I had made my decision to finish but it was not easy. Kenny's problems after all were primarily due to a sudden end of a very close relationship with his father. Sometimes in the sessions I had felt like his father and, although there had been good progress with our work together and I believed that now was a good time to round off our therapeutic relationship, it had been difficult to decide that the sessions should come to an end.

In retrospect, I feel that I was right not to extend the therapy further. One fear that I had was that Kenny's mother might undermine my work in the future. I felt that my warm and inevitable relationship with her son, who never 'shared' with her, would eventually generate some jealousy in her and negate all the good therapeutic work. This can occur despite all the best efforts of the therapist. Another possible effect of too long a duration of therapy can be to make the family too reliant on the clinic, which could be a move from the 'not-so-able' to 'disabled'!

I have found on a number of occasions that the problem of being taken on by some as a replacement for a dead father or grandfather means that I have to be careful not to make my 'exit' another bereavement.

Before we met that day I looked at some of Kenny's earlier creations. The first pieces which I believe initiated positive change in the process were models of hats on women and spots on men's clay faces, which were, Kenny said, bullet holes. He had commented that the woman's moods are known by the hat she wears. This seemed to connect with his mother's moods.

During the next few sessions, Kenny worked through a story about a king in a castle in which was a cage. He drew many scenes and I joined in with him at his request. In Kenny's story, the king comes out of the castle while a woman and a child remain in the cage. The king escapes imprisonment but eventually comes back and frees the woman and child. I could see parallels here concerning his father's death and his mother's state of mind. Perhaps the king leaving the imprisoned woman and child together is understandable but there could be much debate about the return of the king. Understanding the story is happily much less important than its expression and the relief that seems to follow the sharing.

These creations had been followed by Kenny choosing

to make a cardboard 'house' – not a coffin, says Kenny – for his dead hamster. This he did with great care, colourfully papering the inside of the box. At a previous session Kenny had also made a big open pyramid which was to be a house for his cat. He chatted about pharaohs, mummies, Canopic jars and his school visit to the Egyptian Room in the British museum. I chose to point out gently to Kenny the link between the king of former sessions and the pharaoh; both were kings.

The box and the pyramid had been taken home immediately, before they were fully finished. There was no comment from Kenny about kings and pharaohs after the dead hamster's coffin was made; fathers and coffins were never mentioned. It was 'the box', never 'the coffin' for the hamster. Kenny's creations were clearly about his relationship with his parents and his thoughts on death. There was a feeling of urgency in placing them in Kenny's home.

Kenny came brightly into the art room. I greeted him warmly, reminded him that it was his last art therapy appointment and asked what he would like to do. He was friendly and chose to work with clay, which he quietly took from the bin. Kenny had known for some weeks that today we would finish. Impulsively, I said, "I think I'll work in clay, too. I'll make a king." Perhaps I was thinking about Kenny's earlier story and the part that the king had played in it.

Kenny worked at his clay and said, "I'm going to make a canopic box for the spirit."
I was surprised but did not say that canopic boxes, found in ancient Egyptian tombs near to the mummy and containing the body's entrails, are not really for spirits.

Kenny told me that he had seen 'canopic jars' at the museum. "It's to be closed up and kept," he added quietly. He wasn't going to say whose spirit he might be talking about and I had a deep feeling that I should not ask. With great intensity he began to flatten the clay. He rolled it out, cut it up but could not get particular pieces together. Then he asked me to help, which I did. Kenny cut a hole in the centre of the flattened clay.

Next, he made a lid with a strange hanging claw upon it. This was all done with great activity and quiet intensity. Meanwhile, I worked on my little clay king sitting on his throne. Kenny was not interested in my figure and seemed to exclude me for some time, which I felt quite comfortable about. I believed that I should carry on quietly chatting, leaving spaces here and there.

Suddenly, quite spontaneously, Kenny began to tell me almost inaudibly about a dream: "I dreamt about a scarecrow last night. I was going down an alleyway when a man looked out a window – a horrible man. The man is breaking the window and jumping out and running after me. I run and I am scared! Then a scarecrow comes along – not a scarecrow in raggy clothes but in a leather jacket, well dressed. The scarecrow tries to catch up with the bad man. I ran. The scarecrow has a gun but he is trying to get the man who has a bat – a baseball bat – who is trying to attack me. The scarecrow stops the man."

I asked, "Was it a good scarecrow protecting you?" No response. I began to change my clay king into a scarecrow. During this time of talk, both Kenny and I have been working intently on our clay models. Our intensity of focus upon the clay eventually enabled the flow of description. Putting fingers into clay often loosens the tongue, such a valuable thing in therapy!

Eventually from the silence Kenny replied, "Yes, he was protecting me." I said, "Do you feel you need to be protected in real life?" "Sometimes..." Kenny replied, and I felt in the room the enormous sadness of the loss of his father. Quiet again, Kenny continued with the clay canopic box. He found it difficult to make it stand and took lots more clay from the bin. I gently observed,

"Yes, it needs lots more clay to balance it." We both continued quietly with our models.

I decided to break the quietness. "How is that boy now?" I asked, meaning the boy but not emphasising 'him' as being Kenny in the dream story; this gives a comfortable distance. "Am I right in saying he's afraid? He doesn't feel so sad." Kenny replied, "No, I don't feel so sad..." He did not say 'he' as I had.

I remembered fragments of previous talk and said, "Now that the sad feelings are going, we have to look at change! We've decided that, haven't we? You do want to change . . ?" I was referring to Kenny's naughty behaviour. Kenny nodded in agreement. "I'm better in school now and at home sometimes."

I believed that Kenny was trying hard but having worked in schools for so many years, I could imagine that he had such a reputation as a naughty boy that it would take time before any changes were noticed. I did not want to add further comment, which might have spoilt the positive mood; I smiled and focussed a little on my model, adding details to my scarecrow king who sat there happily on his throne. How useful it always is to have these magical images in the room, to have more than discussion.

There seemed to be a powerful energy in the room, with the heavy form of the deathly canopic box near to the scarecrow who was a king upon his throne, apparently ready to protect Kenny.

I asked about Phillip, a boy Kenny had mentioned as being "Always in trouble."
"Sometimes things go wrong at school when you are with Phillip?" Kenny left his clay to stare into space. "Phillip has sad feelings inside, too. Phillip should come to art therapy. I feel better now and Phillip would be better if he came." This was news to me.

"Phillip feels sad?" I queried.

"Yes... Phillip wets his bed, too." This was the only time that Kenny gave away the fact that he would often wet his own bed.

Kenny's whole demeanour spoke of his concern for Phillip and his own anxiety to find a way to change.
I tried to respond but without words. I wanted to show concern but I left the space open for Kenny, so we continued to work the clay within another period of silence. Eventually I enquired, "You say you've not been angry with your mother this week?" knowing that I had changed the subject but I did want some 'mother-thoughts'. Time was running out.

Kenny said, "I used to be angry with her because she killed Dad and I used to kick her." I was surprised by this sudden revelation. Kenny continued quietly but with great intensity: "She should have looked after Dad! She could have! If she looked after Dad, he wouldn't have died!" This was a very moving exclamation, not spoken before. There was a long pause before Kenny added in a more controlled, matter-of-fact tone, "I was angry with her."

I responded, "You were angry with her because your dad died?" Kenny nodded and added, "Yes but now I know really it wasn't her fault, so I've stopped being angry."

Minutes passed and we were absorbed in our modelling. "You were better at home this week?" I enquired.

Kenny nodded again.

"Did you tell your mum what you have told me?"
I asked quietly.

"No... but I will..."

"She may cry but that will be okay. She may be sad and cry because you have been so upset – but not because she's angry with you."

Kenny listened attentively and looked closely at his nearly completed clay box. "I've changed. I've not been the same at home – better!"

Kenny seemed quite anxious to please and was quite insistent that he had changed but he was very busy getting his canopic box right and I had finished modelling my scarecrow. After a while I thought about Kenny's dead hamster.

"Did you bury your hamster?"

"Not properly; he's in the garden. The time isn't right. It has to be done right."

"Yes, it has to have a ceremony, doesn't it? I've got to go to a funeral tomorrow." This was true. "Have you decided on a type?"

"Not yet..."

The room seemed very quiet. After a while I continued, "It would be good to talk to your mum and tell her what you've told me. Would you like to tell her in my office?"

"No, I'll tell her when I go out," Kenny very firmly responded.

Gently, I tried to move him from this position but to no avail. If only Kenny's mother could have shared in Kenny's expressiveness that day – but of course, it is quite unlikely that had she been with us, Kenny would have talked as he did.

Then I needed to tell Kenny that the time was coming to a close and to remind him that this was our last art therapy session. However, I also reminded him that we were good pals and that he could always call in to see me informally.

"You'll need to come back to collect your box when it's dry. You know where I am. Art therapy is finished but I'll expect you to ring me or visit me. Now would you like to get your mum and show her what you've done? Would she like to know how you have changed and are changing?"

"Yes," Kenny surprisingly agreed. At this stage he was relaxed and exuded contentment. A few moments later his mother joined us. Kenny was calm, he was smiling and immediately told his mother how good the session had been and how he was changing. He seemed to be on the point of telling her about his anger towards her since his dad's death but his mother was unhappy and forceful and did not really appear to hear or see her son. She looked at me, not him and told me how much Kenny had been playing up at home.

He instantly changed, looking tense and defensive but his mother continued to complain loudly about her son's behaviour. I gently insisted that she take some notice of Kenny's model and said, "Well, that is all changed now. Kenny now knows why he has been angry. He wants to change and he is going to tell you why things have happened. A lot of his sad feelings have gone! He has changed inside but it may take a little while to change outside, especially as he is known to mess about in school."

I am rarely so confident about a wish to change but confident I was. Kenny nodded to his mother and added that he was at his worst when he was with Phillip. Next, she criticised Phillip at some length! Kenny was then no longer showing the concern for Phillip that he had shown earlier. His mother was not at all interested in our clay models. I realised that she herself was struggling with the loss of her husband. This negative effect of the adult upon the potential for speedy healing of the child is very common. Kenny was adversely affected by his mother's bereaving depression.

As we were at the end of the session and the next patient could be waiting, I did something that I had not done before. I gave Kenny, from my drawer, photo of himself with one of his models that I had taken at an earlier session, a small head of a woman. Kenny seemed pleased but turned away to play with pieces of clay, ignoring his mother. Suddenly he had four little clay 'finger-pots' on his fingers hitting hard against his forehead, strange behaviour. His mother corrected him immediately and loudly.

I then tried to rescue Kenny and make some positive comments about his work over the weeks and his progress. We all then moved into the empty waiting room. I was able to talk to his mother for a short time, to try to help her to recognise the reality of Kenny's desire to change and to acknowledge the importance of listening to what he wanted to say to her. They were, I suggested, both struggling.

I also offered some ideas about his attention-seeking behaviour in the session and what the clay drumming on the forehead might have been about. To me it appeared to symbolise the criticism of his mother 'hitting' him, a kind of hitting his head against a wall. Not so much a feeling of being physically struck but an emotional striking. Kenny's fingertips were not enough to demonstrate this. Heavy clay was required. I gently suggested all of this to Kenny's mother while he was at the window, distracted by cars being parked outside the clinic. Basically she was listening but not clearly perceiving, because of the profound complexity of her distress at what I was saying. I realised of course that the clay fingers explanation was extremely simplified or even incorrect. I was doing my best.

The two models were too fragile to take home that afternoon. When fully dry I would wrap Kenny's box for him. I would keep my 'king' in the art room.

Kenny's grey canopic box, which he did not seem inclined to paint at the end of the session, although he could have done as it was quick-drying clay that required no kiln firing, sat upon the secretary's filing cabinet, with my scarecrow king of the same grey clay next to it. The king was not detailed but had straw-like pieces protruding from its coat and sat in a dignified way. The canopic box was quite neat on its plain surface but had an ill-formed claw upon the lid, which fitted quite well. I had made no decision about what would happen to the king but Kenny settled the matter for me.

In this period I was part-time at the clinic and while I was away Kenny called in with his mother, when she attended counselling with the psychiatrist. He earnestly informed the secretary that he had called to take away his two models and the secretary boxed them up for him. I am confident that the king ended up in the right place, alongside the canopic box. When I last heard of Kenny he was doing well but that was a long time ago.

When I think back over the years, with a clear picture in my mind of the canopic box and the scarecrow king, I am left hoping that the models continued to give Kenny optimism. The single most important moment of the last session, and perhaps the most important of the whole series of sessions, was surely Kenny's disclosure of the reason for his anger. The moment of disclosure may have been 'fixed' to the canopic box as he finished it. For him to consider the box would often bring, I believe, a return to that moment and the disclosure. There had been deep emotion in his voice. I had received this in the safe environment that I had provided. It was received non-judgementally and together we had explored the blaming of his mother.

I had become progressively more aware of Kenny's mother's great difficulty concerning her loss. It is not unusual for a loving parent to say something like, "Fix him and then I'll be okay!" There is much avoidance in this. The child is usually able to move on in bereavement but an adult or adults may be stuck in their progress and, usually without knowing it, in some way hold the child back. It might be that the request should be, "Fix me and he'll be okay," and in this case the mother was being helped by the psychiatrist.

The last session and the home-coming of the clay models had contained all the elements for a satisfactory conclusion to the therapy. Sadly, the inadequate and negative response of Kenny's mother was the stumbling-block. I appreciate how difficult it must have been for her; although something in me would have offered never-ending art therapy for Kenny, I knew this to be wrong. The ending was correct.

Currently I may bring parents with difficulties into such therapeutic art interaction but in this case it was best for me to put my view to the consultant psychiatrist, which I did. She said that it helped her to better counsel Kenny's mother. I do hope that she managed to move on before Kenny lost all the positives he had found within himself in art therapy.

I believe that his memories of his symbolic work without any interpretation will themselves stay to assist him. His imaginings and creations were so very powerful.

Chapter 6

Sam's Story of a Journey

In the 1980s I had the rare opportunity to use art therapy in a busy classroom in a mainstream school. I discussed with the head teacher the possibility of working with a group of children at his school; in a weekly lesson with a class of ten-year-olds I planned to encourage 'free drawing' in such a way that stories, hopefully original, would be produced in picture form. The idea was that the usual priority given to written work would be avoided and an emphasis given to drawing.

I believed that the children would have good feelings about themselves, especially those who were not good at expressing themselves in writing and that the school might be encouraged to include expressive art in the curriculum as a result.

Some expressions of deeper feelings might emerge, I suggested to the head teacher, as is seen in art produced by clients in art therapy. The aims while two-fold – first, to give an opportunity for 'free' narrative drawing and second, to seek evidence of a more profound form of expression – did not include attempts to introduce any therapeutic procedures. It was merely an opportunity to observe and, perhaps, to introduce some friendly forms of discourse with the children to better understand their imaginings. I had hoped to have no more than twelve children in my group – ideally fewer – but in the end the class numbered twenty. There were four weekly sessions, each of an hour's duration.

Evaluation of the project with 'befores' and 'afters' was generally not possible, because there were few 'free' drawings to be found in the school. Most children's drawing was to illustrate their subject, to be placed in their folders and any free drawing, I was told, resulted in those pictures being taken home and, according to some children I asked, soon disposed of!

All considered, however, I found the sessions satisfactory. The girls differed from the boys without exception, in that their subject matter was more gentle. Theirs included domestic scenes, fruit and ideas similar to, or copied from, fairy stories. The boys chose space adventures, violence, wrestling, ghostly castles, skateboarding and cars in collision. Without exception, every boy pursued one or more of these topics. I was quite surprised at that time by the very clear differences in the choices of the sexes.

The girls all began easily; there seemed to have been a recent art lesson using a bowl of fruit as still life and perhaps to please me, a number of colourfully executed pictures of fruit bowls appeared. Many girls were loath to give up this non-narrative mode when I reminded them that our aim was to tell a story. Amusingly, after some gentle encouragement towards a story development, one girl decided to give her still life some unstill-life and the fruit took on faces and moved off, away from the fruit bowl to adventures.

Most children produced a book-form, page to-page progression of pictures. Others simply created a sequence of drawings on separate sheets, while a few drew comic strip styles.

There were two ten-year-old boys who decided not to

co-operate that first afternoon. I discussed the problem with them at the end of the lesson and offered them the opportunity to opt out but they declined. The next week they surprised me with an enthusiastic approach, part of the success being, I believed, because I allowed them to sit together despite their naughtiness the time before.

The taller, Mark, chose a theme which he proposed would be funny. It was along gothic lines, with a cross-section view of a medieval castle with ghost, traps and treasures clearly outlined. The approach was cartoon style and the main influence in his work appeared to come from the Beano and Dandy children's comics.

Mark's story began with the castle and he insisted on writing up a text. The style of his drawing with rigid lines, often ruled, and faces and figures in an effective but clearly derivative comic-book style, never changed. It was a fine piece of work that emerged from the freedom that Mark found and despite the busy environment in which he worked, he concentrated very well. He was proud of his finished 'comic' and his teacher was impressed. Mark achieved something very special and his self-esteem was boosted.

The Story...

Mark's partner in classroom infamy was Sam. Even when trying harder, he was less happy with his drawing, obviously finding it a chore. He took on something of Mark's theme and maintained a comic-book rigidity with frequent use of ruler. From an amusing figure based on a reading scheme character, he moved into rigid portrayals of a man accidentally cutting off his own head. This did not surprise me as nearly all the boys at the end of this particular table were pursuing violent themes. Some were along the lines of medieval fighting, torture and dismemberment, in my experience very usual themes. Indeed, such common graphic descriptions appear to be no more evil than the violent actions of such characters as Bugs Bunny, Donald Duck or Felix the Cat.

At some point, unobserved by myself, Sam took himself off to an empty adjoining classroom with a bundle of papers and began a new story. Each piece of paper was gradually covered by lines and I did observe his busy involvement from a distance but partly by design and also because I was sharing my time with the many children in the class, I did not approach Sam until the end of our final session. He simply came in and worked through the hour and was, to my surprise, quite serious about the whole project.

While Mark's drawings followed a traditional sequence, Sam took a different approach. "They are," Sam said, "what they are." Most of the scenes were of lands visited by his 'people'. They included a somewhat pastoral view, cities and giant machines. Each picture is from a different place, he said; apart from the beginnings of 'the travels' with stars and with the clocks, he was unsure of the sequence and believed that this was not important. A different land (or it seemed to be when he talked of it, mysteriously hidden different planes of existence not easily accessible to ordinary people) was presented on each piece of paper. 'The sorry tv' written upon the screen remains a mystery but at the time I felt that the tv was apologising for its presence.

The beginning of Sam's story was not clearly described and there was, he told me, no ending. His pictures were, to me, the most aesthetic of all the work produced by the children, perhaps because of the freeness of the line. I felt that his emotions made the drawings flow. This quality he dismissed, saying it was "not really good – it's just that I was in a hurry."

These pictures and their sense of mystery were clearly different from his usual rigid style of drawing. I was able to review his drawings, collected in the usual way

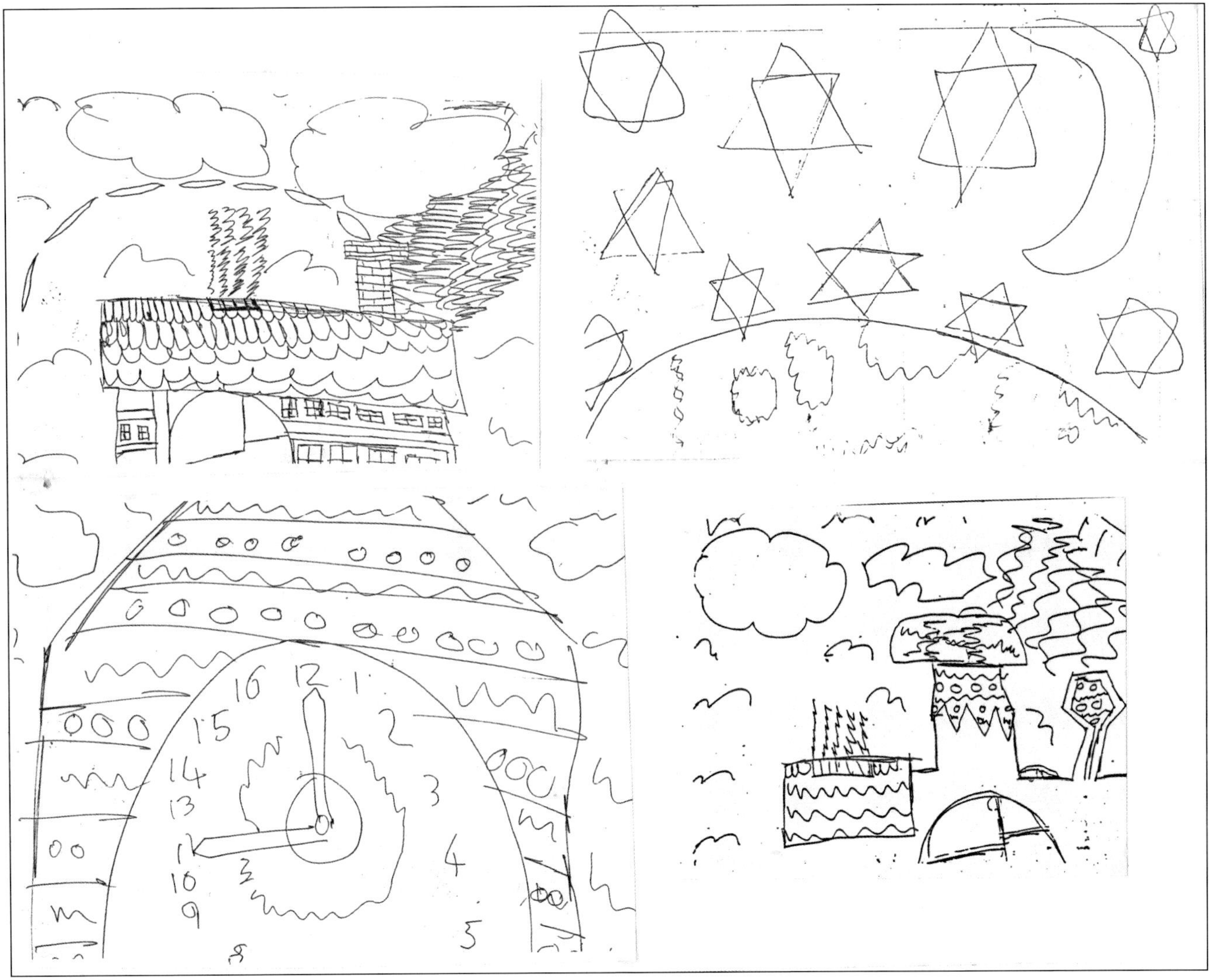

for his folder, over a ten-week period. Because I feel that his project pictures were expressive and differed greatly from his usual work, I propose that the freedoms offered (and perhaps also a good relationship following my very firm but friendly advice after our first session) enabled Sam to enter into a very personal mode of expression. I also believe that when he produced the drawings and then again when he considered their content, deep personal feelings were released.

In particular, it seems that his experience of the death of a loved one, while not easily perceived in his drawings, stimulated and affected this change of expression and style. My opinion comes from what he told me about his drawings when all were finished.

Defining the Story

As planned, I began to interview some of the children about their drawings. Sam was the third. Other children demonstrated quite vivid imaginations and all seemed derivative of at least parts of well-known stories. Each would be of some interest to the reader but I have selected Sam's work here because it is a good example of an unguided and private process of picturing, which expressed deep emotions.

I avoided the clinical interview situation, with a spare classroom and a tape recorder, as potentially intimidating and chose instead an informal chat with scribbled notes. In retrospect and given Sam's response, perhaps he would have been just as expressive with a tape recorder present. What follows is taken from my notes at the time:

Sam: "The story is all my idea. Little people. The dad of all the little people died. He had made a model village for them – met lots of other people. There was a kind of explosion that went round and round. They went into a new place – they were sucked in!"

Later, I asked at what point the father had died and how the young children were. Sam said that the father "died shortly before the tunnel appeared". The children were not simply small because of their youth; they were in fact "midgets".

I asked Sam why stars and music featured in his story. We also see televisions and clocks, which appear to be important. Sam explained, "The music... is when the night comes and they walk into another place because it is night! When it is morning they saw... the massive televisions... pictures... music was just starting."

"Then, 'End!' it says on the television. It doesn't mean the end of the story."

Interestingly, I could find no drawing of a television with 'End' upon it but there is a television with 'The sorry tv' written upon the screen, which remains a mystery. At the time I felt that the tv was apologising for its presence.

After the death of the father and a kind of explosion, the midgets fly down the 'tunnel'. "There were", he said, "those stars when they were sucked in. They could see these things around them. They landed in a place where there were loads of clocks – they struck, it nearly deafened them... they kept moving on... they saw many scenes."

Sam appeared to be coming to the end of his descriptions. He did add that the 'unusual building' was made for the children by the father. This is drawn twice. I had noticed from a distance that these appeared about halfway through Sam's picture making. The tall buildings with lots of windows were the last picture, "not an end to the story," Sam emphasised.

At this point in the interview, my experience told me that I was probably about to be 'dismissed' by Sam, as he had now finished. Although I had not then properly assimilated what he had said, I wanted to return to the death of the father, but I was losing the thread of connection between Sam and myself. I tried gently but Sam was fidgeting and now looking away.

I asked, "Why did the father die?" and Sam replied, "He was old." I had many questions but wished to avoid an interrogation. I said, "Why put that in your story?"
Sam thought for a while. "I guessed it would be better if a man were dying – it makes a story more interesting."
'Well, that's true,' I thought. It appeared that the interview was at an end. Sam's story so far was:

1: A father provides for his midget family, even a special home.
2: He dies.

3: The children are sucked into a tunnel; there are stars.
4: They land, to be faced with noisy clocks. The children are not like their father; they are midgets, small and vulnerable. They see and are nearly deafened by the clocks.
5: They move on in darkness. There is music and there are pictures on great screens. They face writing declaring: 'The End' but it is not really the end. "There is no end, Sam tells me.

As it turned out, Sam was not finished with me, merely looking about him, fidgeting and really wishing to leave. Then he suddenly became re-animated. I believe he decided to 'own up' about the inclusion of death in his story. As he had said, death is certainly dramatic and good story telling, but a death in the family seemed to have given him the idea.

Sam spoke deliberately, expressing himself well: "My cousin's mum died about a month before this story. There is a picture of her on our wall at home. I looked at it and it gave me an idea. Something else gave me an idea! I've only got one Nan left! When my cousin's mum died, my mum and my cousin's kept it to themselves. They didn't want me to be upset."

I asked Sam whether he was in fact much upset by this loss. Was he very fond of her? Did he know her well? He responded almost defiantly, "No!" He did not know her well. She was not special to him, in any way. I thought that he protested too much.

We paused. Sam continued, "I didn't know. They moved stuff from that house to our house... like cabinets and furniture. She was old. It was a special place I used to visit. Three days a week."

I felt that Sam really was fond of his aunt. I missed some of his words and then he seemed a little confused and made some vague comments, which briefly interrupted what had been a commanding flow. He said that he had actually called to see her but she wasn't there. He took a deep breath and plunged back into his clear descriptions:
"I guessed! They only told me later... it made my throat feel funny. Now I'm over it."

He paused, looking absently out of the window. "I was over it... went on my bike to see where she was buried... then I felt bad again... It took longer to get over it."

Sam became quiet and it was time for class changes. Some children started to arrive and Sam said that he was off. I thanked him and we parted company. He seemed happy enough, despite his story of bereavement. At one point he had said that his drawings were "not sad".

The end of the interview with Sam convinced me that, even if the pictures had not been intended to tell the story exactly as the boy now described it, what they expressed concerned death.

Possibly the unusual flow and expressiveness of the drawings were triggered by the thoughts of his recent bereavement. Certainly he was disturbed by this loss and in particular by the fact that he suspected the loss and confirmed it before his parents told him of it. The opportunities afforded in our sessions enabled him to express and consider his feelings in a positive way.

The process of communication might be seen like this:

1: An initial reticence to participate in free narrative drawing.
2: Encouragement.
3. A flow of drawings devoid of human figures ("I can't do people properly.")
4: A verbal description by Sam of his story.
5. A separate story explaining how a death gave him the idea of including death in his verbal and drawn narrative.

This total process of expression by Sam leads me to suppose that a very personal consideration of death is contained within it. I also suppose that, consciously or unconsciously, some or all of the drawings are images concerning the following:
Life – the beginning, the family, the house and acquaintances; the delicacy of life – the midgets needing care and provision; the death, near-death experience, or even a memory of birth experience – being drawn along the tunnel, the stars and the planet; the reality of ageing/time – the clocks; death as non-ending (Sam had supposed that he had written 'the End' on a tv screen but had instead written 'The Sorry television' instead. Sorry about death, or about time and life passing?) He later said that the last picture was not the end.

There is certainly an expression of feeling concerning one death within the family.

He added that he had only one grandmother remaining. It seemed that within the drawing and chatting Sam was in the broadest sense considering his current feelings about death and perhaps at the same time life, birth and even re-birth.

It is perhaps impossible to ascertain how original the complete narrative is. I asked Sam whether he had seen the old science fiction tv series, Time Tunnel. He had but that, he maintained, had nothing to do with his story. In this American television fiction people moved into a different time by walking down a vertical metallic tunnel decorated with ringed black stripes. There are no stars or planetary curve visible in this presentation. Sam's idea is, in fact, much nearer to the near-death experiences recorded in the researches of, amongst others, Dr Raymond Moody and Dr Michael Sabom, where there is seemingly an out-of-body experience of floating along a dark tunnel into an inviting light area.

There is a feeling of space being transversed and sometimes some star and/or planetary indications in these visions. I asked Sam whether he had seen any recent television programmes about 'death experiences'. He looked confused, perhaps wondering what I was talking about. He had not. He was, however, following the television science fictions series, 'Land of the Giants'. In these stories we follow the adventures of early space voyagers on a planet of giant humans. Sam said that he did not base his idea of midgets on this. "It's quite different!" he emphasised with some annoyance!

It can't be proved that Sam's series of drawings or the interview that followed, with the exception of 'funny throat' feelings and 'getting over it', are expressions of the child's very deep feelings regarding death. I do believe, though, that his 'art opportunity' came at the right place and the right time. Sam had a chance, not usually allowed in mainstream education, to express personal feelings in a useful way – and he took it. It was also interesting to see that the boy produced a more fluent style of drawing than hitherto. Sam used his imagination (without the limitations of the written word) to produce something of significance.

If the idea of travel after death by floating along a tunnel had not been taken by Sam from the media or from adults, it is interesting to consider how he might have arrived at such imagery.

The significance of the drawings is that their production made it possible for Sam to express feelings concerning life and death. I believe that his narrative and drawing expressions relating to this matter are a useful manifestation of his concerns and ideas, which he will no doubt remember, consider and re-consider as he evolves towards a healthy response to bereavement. He was externalising some deeply felt concepts. There is an indication that Sam's parents should not have avoided telling him of their loss. It would seem that Sam was making some sense of death and life by turning to a pictorial communication to himself from himself, as if he felt that such ideas could not be shared with his family. This is frequently seen in processes of art therapy.

Looking back, I still find this a very powerful story. It is very unusual in that this comes from group work and not from the privacy of a one-to-one session. It shows the power of imagery. Although I cannot prove it in this case, I believe that it brought comfort to Sam.

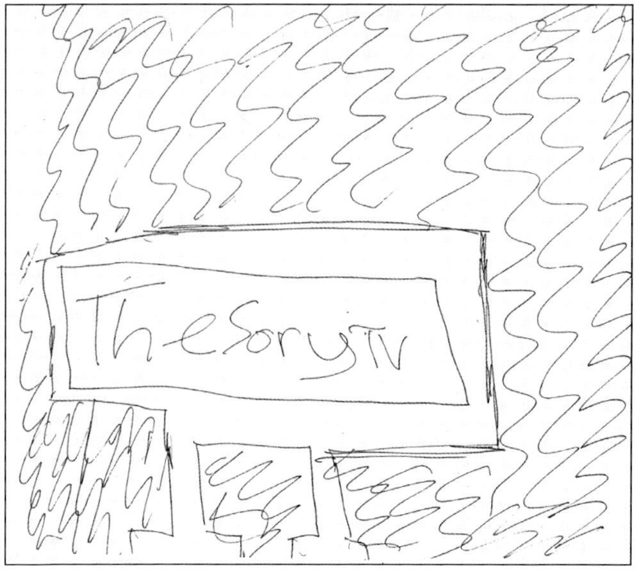

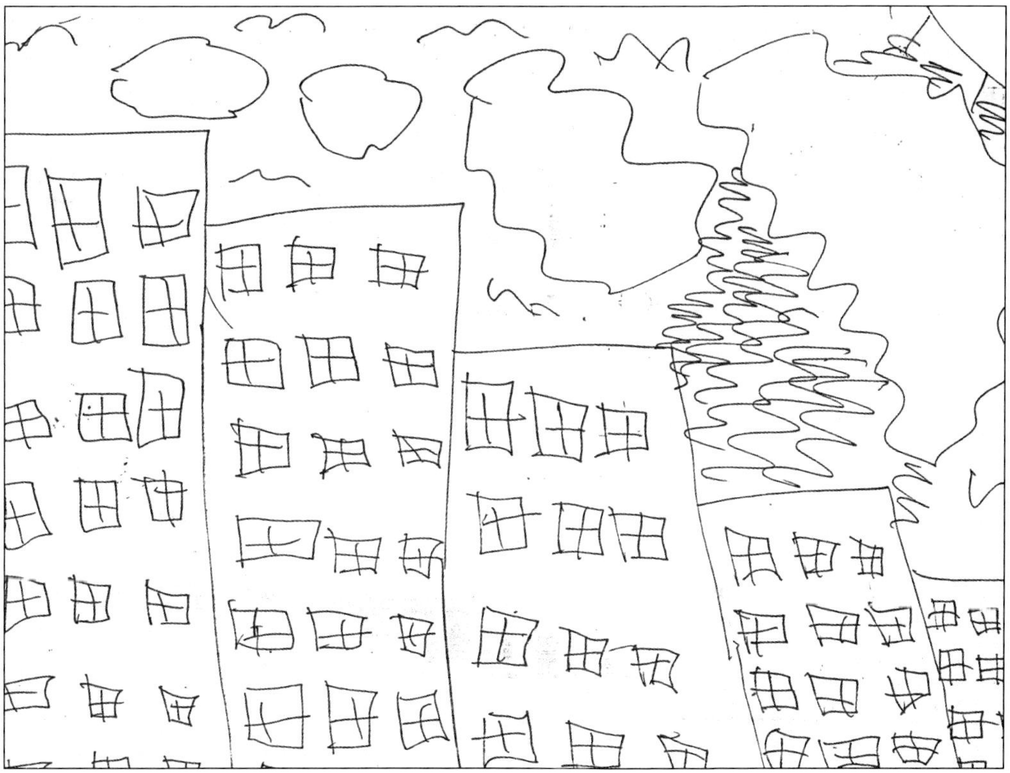

Chapter 7

Bella's Wisdom

Bella was eight years of age. She had been very naughty, easily upset, throwing lots of temper tantrums and wetting the bed. Colleagues in the Department of Child and Adolescent Psychiatry had advised Bella's parents on better techniques for handling her behaviour. She was clearly still upset by earlier conflicts, now resolved, between her parents. Two years earlier, they had split up for a time and she had not seen much of her father. Matters improved and her parents were happily re-united but Bella's deteriorating behaviour did not change for the better.

With the clinic's support and advice the problems began to diminish. Latterly it was thought that art therapy might help. Given the opportunity Bella drew and painted which left a relaxed little girl, according to her parents, after each weekly session. It was not easy to connect her artwork with her situation but her behaviour improved even more as the prescribed five appointments were attended.

At the last session Bella looked at a drawing of a castle she had chosen to create during the previous appointment. She asked me to write down a story of a king and queen who lived in the castle, which gave her tremendous satisfaction and seemed very much to connect with her mother and father.

Bella's story of the king and queen, as spoken while looking at her castle picture

"The king is in the tunnel. He is watching the rain.

"It is raining and the king gets wet,
His hair gets wet, cos the crown's got holes in it
(crowns are like that!)
The queen warned him but he didn't listen!
Kings never listen!
Now he thinks that he shouldn't
Have gone out in the first place,
Not just walked out of the door.

"The king and queen are getting married tomorrow
On a Thursday.
Later they die on a Thursday.
This is so that everyone will know that
Thursday is their special day."

What a wonderful story. Bella was so very proud of her 'castle and royal family' pictures and the story. As she had requested, she took all of her work home and all was exhibited proudly on the kitchen wall, including the story which I had typed up.

Although I did not enquire when I met with her parents, as Bella took the story and the castle picture home, they did give me knowing smiles and seemed at least to guess that the king and queen were Mummy and Daddy.

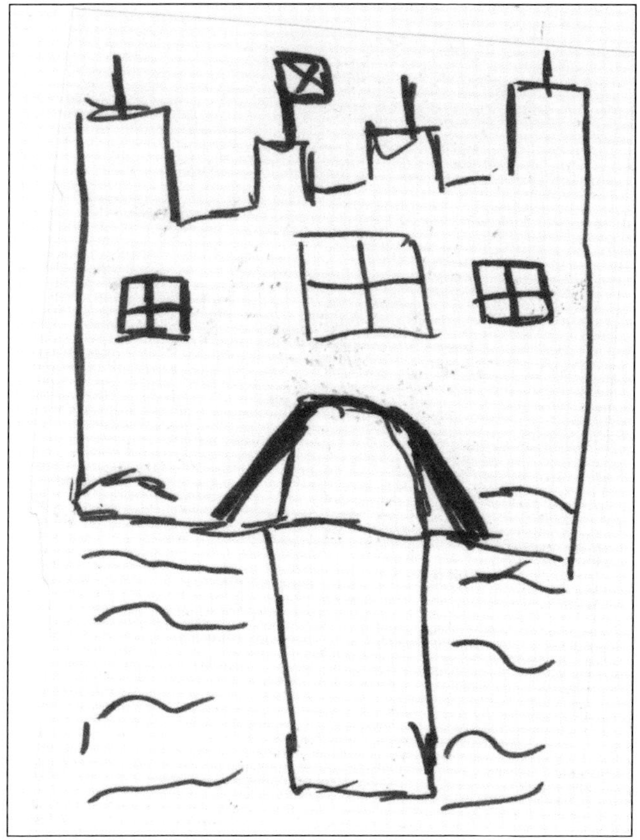

Although I say that it is important not to impose one's own personal interpretation on a patient's work while in progress, it can sometimes be useful to draw conclusions in retrospect.

Here I think – although there is every possibility that I am wrong - that the king 'in the tunnel' might be an unhappy or even depressed Daddy (as perhaps he was at the time of the separation). Next, in the rain, he gets wet; his royal crown and kingly status are of little use. His wife can say, "I told you so!" and he is choosing not to hear her. The king-like Daddy 'walked out of the door', which he now regrets.

Why the importance of Thursday? Perhaps this is a magical bond making a special togetherness. Neither Bella nor her parents gave any clues to the Thursday phenomenon. Whether or not Thursday was significant there is a feeling for me that this is a 'grounding'. It is as if within this fantasy there is a need for reality. There is a togetherness for these parents in their marriage and eventually they are still together in death. Whether we understand the metaphors, which are surely there, or not, we can enjoy the many facets of this story.

I like to think that the little exhibition continued to exert a positive influence on the mother and father as much as on Bella the creator. A year later, I met up with the parents by chance and they told me how well the family was doing.

Chapter 8

Using Art to Improve Communication

Many summers ago, when I was working in an educational setting in Norway, I shared paper and crayons and even, to my surprise, feelings with a mature Norwegian lady who, because my voice reminded her of her abusive father, was too nervous of my presence to work with me. As she had little English and my Norwegian is non-existent, I asked the rest of the group to suggest to this lady that she and I might draw and doodle silently together on a great sheet of paper spread upon the floor. We soon laughed, exclaimed and gestured as we played with paint and crayons. The problem was soon solved, we related and communicated well (perhaps as toddlers would!) without words. It was not long before she tolerated my gruff vocals. If this really did add up to a sizeable and very natural breadth of communication, why should 'art-communication' be left to art specialists?

How usually effective is such 'communication'? I have had the luxury of spending two long periods of secondment, in which in the first instance I researched the drawing development of multi-handicapped children and in the second instance the drawing development of 'normal' children from one to five. It became clear that even with the youngest (in mind and/or body) to make a mark on a surface and to consider the mark was of great importance. The pencil or crayon used to mark was surprisingly rarely sucked or chewed. Abstract, much loved drawn patterns are constantly reproduced. I called these unusual and very personal patterns "favoured configurations". Contrary to conclusions reached through previous research, these abstracts develop alongside the more socially acceptable representational picturing (usually of "me", "Mummy", Daddy" and later "house").

It does appear that as adults we continue with our abstract pattern production when much conscious effort is made listening or speaking, for example using the telephone or attending a lecture. These we call our doodles and they are clearly very personal. Given the luxury of a few years at art school we would no doubt eventually decide, and I mean this quite seriously, to either develop our 'doodle sense' of marking the canvas, pursue 'picturing', or even perhaps combine something from both. It does happen.

Really free drawing from young or old is valuable and currently rarely seen in schools. I am not, however, suggesting that such free drawing should, or even can be, dissected and analysed. What I am saying is that free drawing can help relax and help communication. The picturing ability that we develop is the drawing skill that leads to the writing skill, just as historically writing has developed from drawing. The doodling ability can, I believe, contain much more, even very deep, expression. While such patterns express much to the creator, especially perhaps to the child (who is still part-functioning at pre-verbal levels), however, we can only share in such expression through clues. These clues come primarily from speech but also from gaze, expression and gesture. Immersion in considerations of abstract patterns and symbolisms is for the trained therapist and not for those more generally involved.

Why do we not always provide pencils and paper in a 'communication setting'? Perhaps we, not the person who is joining us, lack the confidence to participate in doodling and drawing?

What am I saying here? I am saying that amongst other things, problems – and feelings about these problems – can be better understood when paper and pencil are readily available. Suppose that you are the person seeking better understanding of the person before you. If you yourself are happy to doodle on your paper, as well as the one you are wishing to communicate with, it may be that new avenues of communication open up. It would be a good idea, I think, for GPs to try such approaches and particularly useful within the four-to seventeen-year age range.

Your friendly encouragement and discussion about, for instance, what 'you' and 'I' like to draw and even sometimes 'why' will be useful. We need, "Let's do some scribbles about this," but we do not need to ask "What is it you've drawn?" in such a situation, "Can we talk about what we've drawn?" is more appopriate. We require no analysis but we do need discussion.

I must emphasise that here I am not describing art therapy but art aiding communication. The professional will not, I hope, think of him/herself as a psychologist, psychiatrist or psychotherapist. My function, for instance, as an art therapist is an *enabler*, so that my client can present images and abstractions to him/herself for consideration. This frequently becomes an ongoing process of discovery and better understanding which is truly psychotherapeutic.

My skills have to be diverse and while not always knowing from moment to moment what best to do, I certainly know what I must not do. Art therapy is something very special and I am not suggesting that doctors and others should dabble with it. What I am suggesting is that art (or just drawing, image making or doodling) can lead to useful discussion, especially when dealing with children. Such discussion – though not interrogation – can improve communication and I am sure that this would usually be useful, remedial and, ultimately, time saving.

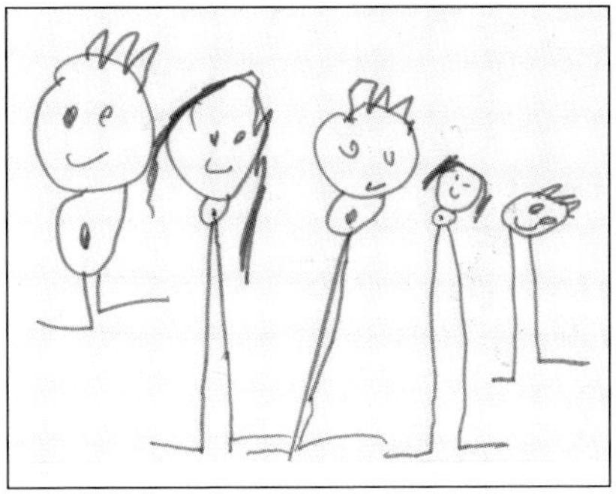

If someone is ill because of stress, it helps to know where that stress is really coming from. While drawing and doodling might not on their own reveal the origin, it is likely that the relaxed situation will open up some better understanding.

All in all, I believe that drawing, painting and modelling, (which does not have to be clay but can be plasticine or even blu-tac), even without the presence of a therapist, can be very relaxing and assist communication; however, too many questions and attempts to analyse the product will easily destroy the process. Carers, members of a patient's family and occasionally friends have asked me how they can continue the art therapy work outside the clinic. Although the enquirers are well-meaning, I usually turn to my peripheral therapeutic knowledge and give 'social-psychological' advice on how best to relate to the patient, rather than 'how to be an art therapist'.

I also, when appropriate, turn to my hospital colleagues for practical advice, which is usually about making the needy person feel at ease and more confident, and generally accentuating the positive and diminishing the negative. Easy advice to carers is to encourage and support good hobbies. Just sometimes that hobby or potential hobby is painting! But I warn of the dangers of interpretation; enthusiastic encouragement from the helper is good enough.

Sharing

In the late Seventies, I was deputy principal and then acting principal at what was then The Spastics Society's largest residential school. My busy schedule always had room in it for me to share the children's art, even in my off duty hours. John, severely affected by cerebral palsy, saw me in the hallway and approached me in his wheelchair. He asked me in his stuttering speech whether I'd like to see some new pictures. I was aware that for some reason he wanted to stay at school in the holidays, and hoped he might give some indication of why he was not looking forward to going home.

We spread his two drawings over my office table and I guessed that they represented the road accident that damaged John's brain and caused his disability. The following is an abbreviated version of our conversation, which I was able to tape-record.

Trevor: John, you're quite an artist; you've done two pictures. There's a lot in them. I think I know what's happening but I might be wrong. Is this a man crossing the road?
John: No
Trevor: It's you who is crossing the road?
John: Yes, here comes the car. I wasn't looking. (My guess is correct) My mummy and daddy were crying.
Trevor: Why?
John: Because I got knocked down.
Trevor: Did you see them?
John: They picked me up.
Trevor: Have mummy and daddy told you about this?
John: Yes
Trevor: But you remember anyway?
John: Yes
Trevor: That was before you were knocked over by the car?
John: Yes... (He panics and mumbles a little)
Trevor: The other picture. You tell me about that one.
John: That's me. The car that knocked me down is here. This is the ambulance.
Trevor: How old were you when this happened?
John: Only three
Trevor: How old are you now?
John: Thirteen
Trevor: Have mummy and daddy told you about the accident? Have they talked about it?
John: No. I remember before the car crash. I know what it is like to be knocked over. I had blood down my leg... I want to stay here at school till I get better.
Trevor: Well, you can stay here. But even if you have a poorly leg, can't you go out?
John: No. My mummy and daddy want to take me to the seaside after I go home.
Trevor: Don't you want to go to the seaside?
John: They can't afford to take me.
Trevor: Who said so? Or do you just think so?
John: I just think so.
Trevor: Why don't you want to go?
John: I don't know.
Trevor: Is it the money? I don't think it's the money.
John: They can't afford to take me to the seaside.
Trevor: That is what you think? They didn't say that, did they?
John: Daddy will have to push me in a wheelchair all the time, won't he? (John's eyes are brimful with tears)
Trevor: Now listen. Let's get this straight. It's not that you are really worried about the money; it's because you will be in a wheelchair, is that it?
John: Yes
Trevor: I see. You didn't tell me that at first, did you?
John: No
Trevor: You're worried about that, are you?
John: Yes
Trevor: Perhaps they don't mind. It will be fun.
John: They've bought a car.
Trevor: You were telling me about them pushing you in a wheelchair.
John: Why did I get knocked over? (We stop a while as John weeps)
Trevor begins again, very gently:

Trevor: You were telling me a little secret. You were telling me that you were worried about your holiday and that they don't want to push you in your wheelchair. Why do you think it will be a nuisance for them to push you in a wheelchair? Don't you think the children will like helping? You tell me.
John: I can't walk.
Trevor: So you really want to walk when you are on holiday. That's what you mean?
John: I want to walk but when I try I fall over.
Trevor: If you go on holiday, it will make everyone happy. They want you to go on holiday. I know you want to walk but they'll be sad if you don't go. Do you think they want you to go?
John: (Thinks for a while and then speaks) Don't know.
Trevor: I'll write and ask them. If they say they really want you to go to make them happy, would you go, even though you can't walk very well?
John: Can I walk?
Trevor: You're doing your best to walk, aren't you?
John: That's what they tell me.
Trevor: You know that's true. Let's think about it. You don't want to go on holiday, because you think it will cost a lot of money. You told me you don't want to go on holiday because they don't like pushing a wheelchair. You told me you don't want to go on holiday because you want to walk and not use a wheelchair. But we know that cannot be, don't we? So why don't you go on holiday, use your wheelchair and walk when you can? Use your wheelchair when you have to. You do your best and make them happy.
John: They can't take my walker. It's too big for the car.
Trevor: Perhaps your mummy and daddy could take a folding walker. You won't need it all the time.
John: But they haven't got a car (even though he said earlier that his parents had bought a car).
Trevor: I see... I wonder if we can send the walker on the train to where you are going. Shall I find out what can be done?
John: Yes
Trevor: I don't believe it's as bad as you think. I think we can get your walker on holiday.
John: I want to stay here for a long time. I can't walk by myself.
Trevor: Will you go on holiday?
John: No
Trevor: How about me and you talking about it tomorrow? I might write to Mummy and Daddy and ask them about your holiday, if you don't mind. How about that?
John: Yes

In this case, the message in the simple drawings was amplified by the child and conversation about them helped to externalise his anxieties. John's ability to draw his accident helped him to discuss his problems. The words from the tape recording speak for themselves. John was asking through his drawings for help. His ability to draw, rather than scribble, allowed him to communicate his fears and this helped us to help him.

Together, John and I composed a letter to his parents so that they could confirm my feelings that his holiday worries were unfounded. Their reply was most helpful and John eventually went happily off on his holidays, with a folding walker from the physiotherapy department. As for John's yearning to be normal, no miracle would be forthcoming but he continued to make progress and to come to terms with his limitations.

I was not then an art therapist; it was just a matter of art helping communication.

The following story of Julie and her Butterflies describes a similar situation, where this time psychiatrist and art therapist combine their skills.

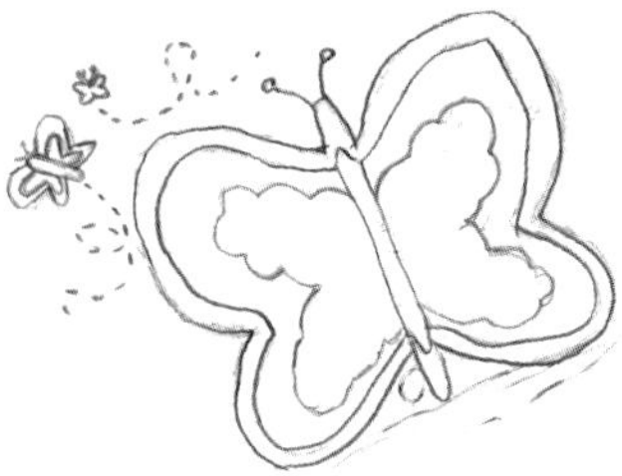

Chapter 9

Julie's Butterflies

While many consultations take time before children can find a way to express themselves and explore what is troubling them through the pictures they produce, on other occasions the breakthrough can be surprisingly swift.

Julie was a case in point. When she came to me she was a withdrawn and bad-tempered, golden-haired six-year-old. She had been regularly rejected by her depressed mother, leading sometimes to her being placed in care. Little real bonding had taken place between Julie and her mother but her parent had begun to make some progress through therapeutic sessions with her psychiatrist, a colleague of mine.

Julie was just starting art therapy and, upon reading her notes, I wondered amongst other things how sympathetic she was to her mother's problems. Certainly, she was very affected by them, as her behaviour showed. Her pictures were to answer my question and were a touching example of the power of metaphor.

In her very first session and after twenty minutes of painting a very stylised, infantile scene with figure, house and flowers which she clearly did not want to talk about, Julie began a new little picture of two butterflies for me. She pointed to the dark red little butterfly. "The little one is a girl, Kate," she told me. "The butterfly lives in a little house... the mother butterfly, the blue one, is Kelly."

The names misled me momentarily, as they did not seem appropriate. Then Julie seemed to tense and she sat upright and spoke in a stumbling way, as if talking to the picture: "Mummy doesn't... like the little one... No!" She paused and shook her head. "The mummy does... yes... like the little one... yes."

Julie stopped and added a letter 'g', which she crossed out and then wrote 'girl'. She sat there, looking still and lost. Understandably, at six years old, she was unused to talking about her problems and just sat there, intently studying the butterflies. Then, with just a minute to go before our session was due to end, Julie beckoned me closer and whispered in my ear: "Baby one doesn't know much about the mummy one!"

The sessions that followed provided the opportunity for a useful dialogue to develop between Julie and myself about her family of adventuring butterflies. She became quite a chatterbox. I never needed to discuss her own situation but only the situation that the two butterflies found themselves in. As the two butterflies played out her various concerns and fears, Julie developed an understanding of her relationship with her mother. She became less angry and her disturbed nights became a thing of the past.

Happily, Julie's mother's psychiatrist was able to feed back, in a very positive way, Julie's Butterfly story to her mother (who was already making progress). In this way, Julie's imagination helped both herself and her mother.

Of course, this situation was much helped by the parallel work of psychiatrist and art therapist. I have often worked in this way with fellow therapists within our department, effectively sharing the cases.

Chapter 10

Some Comments on Art Therapy and Emotionally Disturbed Children

After the 9/11 disaster, there was a call on the internet to all therapists working with disturbed children to forward ideas to New York. This was what I sent. In it I summarised my approach to the subject on one A4 sheet:

It is usually useful to encourage children to play with art materials and produce work. But this process of such art-play even without the product is helpful to the child; it is sometimes relaxing, often calming and always a very basic learning situation. So process is possible just by an adult supplying and encouraging. 'Doing' is the therapy when a child is deeply distressed.

Arguably the 'product' is less useful! Certainly 'product' is the thing that attracts the adult and such interaction can be quite negative: "What is that?" "Perhaps you could add..." "You could do it like this!" even "That's nice!" (When it's not supposed to be nice) etc. Hopefully an experienced art therapist treats product with great respect.

I would say let the kids do what they will with materials. Free process and free product. Let them talk about what they are doing, because in verbal response to their art-play they add great therapeutic value. Art allows expression and to this much more is added when there is 'projection'. (The artist has extra ideas to 'hang' onto the art work.) Let them 'do', then let them focus upon product. Encourage them to talk. Go for, "Could you tell me something about this?" or "Is there a story to this?" Don't ask, "What is it?" Be careful. Trust the process and product and don't muddy the waters with your own interpretation.

If expression and projection is all very painful for the child expect metaphor. Working with, say, dragons rather than say, aircraft is less painful. It's all at arm's length (and more) in metaphor. Wonder what the magical king (that is the Magical King invented by the young artist) is doing but don't let the child be the magical king without that idea coming from the child. Believe me the dragon and the magical king picture/story can bring sensible order to the disordered world of the child as a gift from his/her imagination, much better than an adult's discussion about, for example, aircraft and the President!

So that's it! Let the kids work, listen to them but don't project yourself into their work.

Another idea. Sometimes even in metaphor the product will be too painful. If you, the adult, feel that the child is not 'expressing' ask him/her what you might draw. The child may, while playing with materials or even picturing, project a theme to you which is too painful, even in metaphor/fantasy for them. Of course the adult has to be entirely led by the child (easier said than done). Beware of changing the idea... It must be the child's story. Ask if you are doing the picture correctly. Ask what comes next. Ask if there is a follow-up picture. Summarise the story together as this focuses the power.

Sessions should not be too long – about 40 minutes or so. You can adapt your work to suit groups, perhaps up to 20. And of course children teach us that important things happen at fun times. Even if deep down this is serious business there will be no real flow of ideas without fun being present.

Good luck... Trevor.

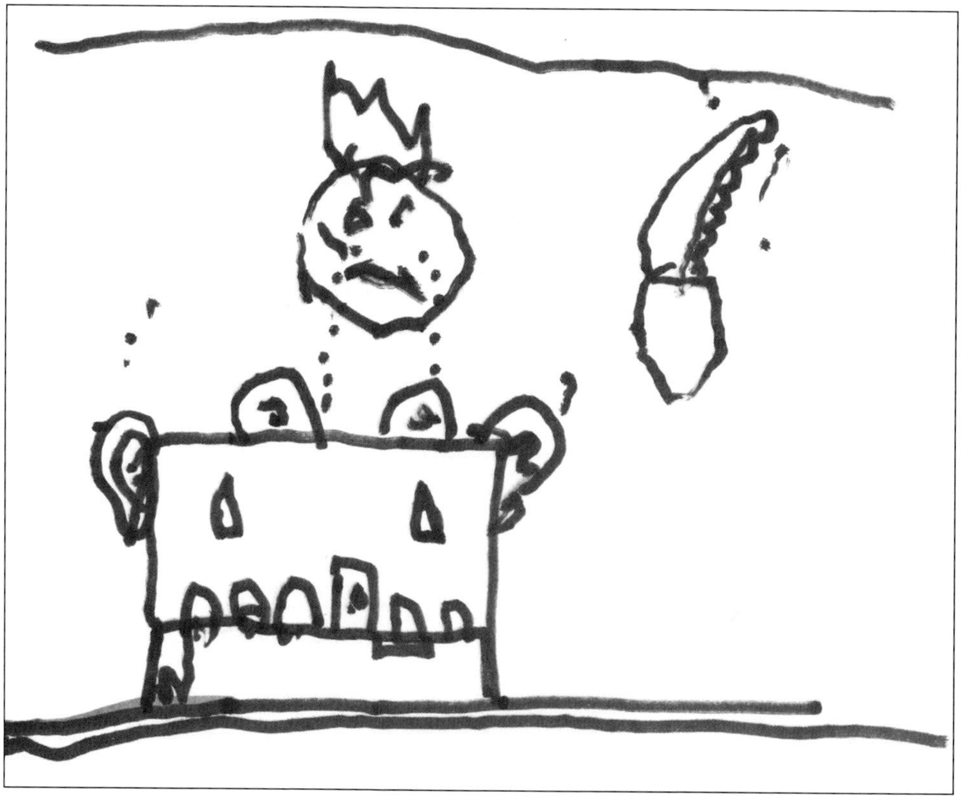

Chapter 11

Theorising About the Artwork, a Painting by an Anorexic Teenager

While I would insist that an 'interpretation' of a picture often brings negatives to the process of therapy (I referred to this earlier) it is clear that even if the client cannot explain what has been created, there is a 'feeling' emanating from the artwork. With both therapist and artist different levels of perception will be occurring. The client, however, verbalising feelings accompanying the image, can give some clarifications to the therapist. The sharing is part of the therapy. The creator must tell the tale, not the therapist!

Within all of this the art therapist will be having feelings about the image and, while not making any formal interpretation, should be helped by this feeling to respond positively to the client. The therapist must be very much aware of the whole environment and what is occurring: the 'feeling' of the space (the room), the physical relationship (for example, how the two people are sitting/standing, body language, facial expressions and tone of voice) and, of course, the 'image'. The image contributes to an overall feeling, so it must be allowed to have its effect upon the relationship. Although the client may 'interpret', the therapist does not need to but is, nevertheless, being aided by his/her perception of that image. It may become, even if temporarily, an inspiration.

The creator may be bringing more and more to his or her creation, both during its creation and after its completion, by interpreting what appears to be in the work. What seems to be happening here is that both the conscious and subconscious are seeing what they need to see. This process of very personal perception (which can also occur when one looks at a flame, a cloud, an ink-blot, etc) is called projection. The therapist is, of course, also projecting and has to be aware of their personal 'projective perception', which can differ greatly from that of the creator.

Sometimes, when there has been good progress and that progress seems to have depended on the images, neither the client nor the art therapist can be sure of what occurred. The therapist needs to be comfortable with such a mystery; to be content with the remediation, or effectiveness of the work.

So, if I am saying that I should not 'define' the image for the artist, as to do so would limit its powerful ambiguity and flexibility of metaphor, what should, ideally, be occurring in the therapy sessions? It seems to me that the most useful perception of and response to the artwork would contain, for the good therapist, a blend of sensitivity, experience, intelligence and that special something that contains these and more – intuition. The therapist has to 'feel' something from the art product, perhaps even unknowingly using infantile mental responses; those feelings and sensitivities that are deep within our minds, connected with early and even pre-language thought processes. Such elements are surely part of intuition.

After the session there is a secondary situation where the therapist may be left alone with the image; the trio becomes a duet. A new feeling. For the therapist the input of the isolated image brings more help of an almost indefinable nature. The empathy may then increase or just change its style. So it is that even without an analysis, the power of the image continues. Of course when the client returns to the therapist and to the image, there will be a difference. That difference can be a very good step forward. In some, but not all cases, the image may end up upon the wall in the artist's home, to 'give off' more positives. This is of course a mixture of seeing what the artist created at the moment of the image's 'birth' and the current emotional state of the artist; what he or she is projecting at the time into the work. The therapy may even continue in this way after the sessions have concluded.

I should add here that we must not take it for granted that the painting, or model, has to appear at the following session. It could wait on the shelf. The artist's need, or the therapist's intuition, will or will not, bring it to the table.

The Painting

I reproduce here the painting 'No Entry'. Unsurprisingly all those years ago, I had strong feelings as I watched the painting develop. It was given to me as a gift by the friendly female artist, so extra to the notes I had to make in the file after that particular session, I could take the time at a later date to collect my thoughts concerning 'No Entry'.

If we look at the painting it gives us a good opportunity to theorise about "meaning".

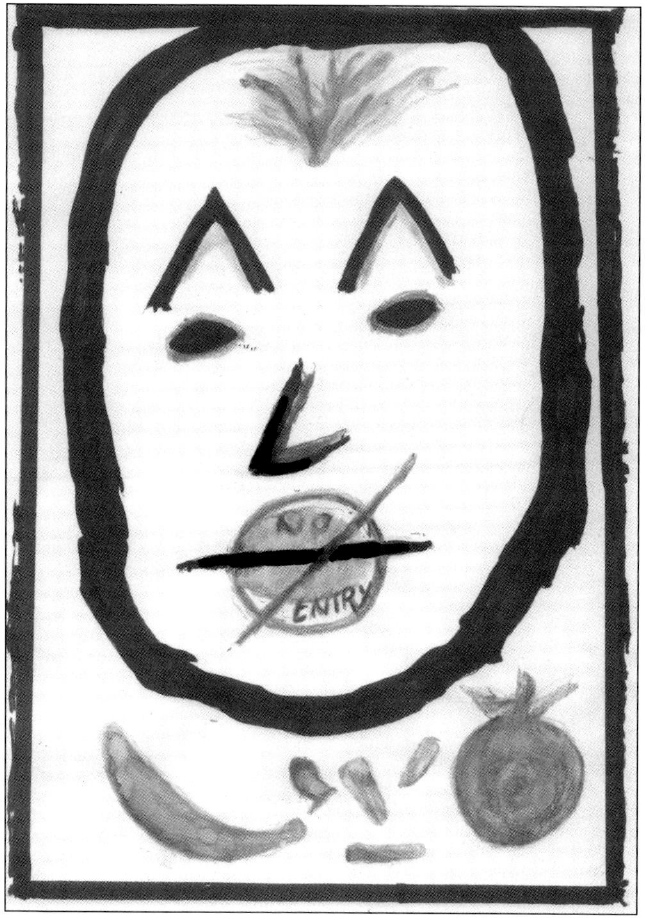

'No Entry'

Unsurprisingly it was created by an anorexic teenage girl when I asked her to paint "just anything" in our first session. I did not ask her about her problems, merely encouraging her painting in a friendly way. She made no "relevant" comments about her picture. She joked about it being "a weird painting" and I was told smilingly, "You can keep it, Trevor."

It can be so misleading to respond to the most obvious part of a therapy picture, in this case the food and the "No Entry" mouth. A sealed lipped face, in my opinion, might well have been made to impress or even satisfy me. She knew that I knew of her anorexia. What might I need from her? Did she think I needed this image? Quite possibly. She was a very nice girl! So we should see what feelings might be hidden in this face. We can look beyond the "no entry" mouth. Even if the picture might be more about thinking than feeling, somewhere we would expect to find emotional expression within it.

For me the powerful black circle of the face is very serious and dramatic, even and perhaps especially when it is considered in isolation. A black rainbow in my mind. It hits or hangs from the top edge of the paper, or so it seems. It can be a deadly black. Of course, black does not have to be deadly. The visually impaired often, I have seen, enjoy black because of its extra clarity. Perhaps the black paint was simply near to the brush? Perhaps the black paint comes first in the manner of "a beginning in drawing" before any coloured filling in. Alone. But also the black gives me a deathly feeling. Despite my experience of alternatives and the possibility of too simple an explanation, that is the strong feeling it gives me. Deathly. Even a coarse rope noose? At least a sadness.

Next, the pyramid or mountain-like eyebrows hold my attention. The nose is a similar shape. Once again blackness, black lines. I feel a sharpness in these shapes. (The artist was a self-harmer.) The accompanying watery blues and greens add to these black lines, bringing a coldness. The most upsetting parts of the picture are, for me, the black eye shapes. So many people have painted in my presence dark holes which they have said they cannot get out of. These red-rimmed black holes are so sad.

I have to remember that in all of this I may be so incorrect but I must allow an overall feeling to touch my heart to help my patient. These 'possibilities' were not shared with the girl but I did ask her how she felt *and* how she felt about the picture even though, as I guessed that she would, she smilingly replied, "I'm fine... the picture is weird," not wishing to say much more.

Before this I had already begun to feel very sympathetic towards her as I watched her choose her colours and paint the face. She was clearly intensely emotionally involved in its production, with fleeting frowns and silent mouthings quickly replaced by 'happy-go-lucky' glances at me and final smiles. Her face looked like a happy face but the face on the paper was nearer the truth; a very sad face.

To me the furrowed forehead in the picture is most unusual, never before seen in a picture produced in my little art room. My response to the red lines is a supposition about angry-feelings. First perhaps the wire-like quality that I see is irritating and angry. Irritation is much the same as anger. Second, and this is due to my experience in art therapy, I had felt that the eyebrows could be mountains or even volcanoes. I saw then that perhaps the 'forehead/anger/irritation' might be a strange sort of disconnected volcanic eruption. Could this be her disconnection from deeper feelings? Sharp, irritating black forehead-mountains disconnecting from an erupting anger?

Over more than forty years I have been told by my patients that their models or paintings of erupting volcanoes were about anger. Many had water, ice or magical devices brought in to cool the heat of anger. One bright ten-year-old boy once told me, "See that exploding volcano? That is my anger and my big sadness... which is kind of the same thing, you know!" It is good to deal with the volcano.

So it is, then that this painting expresses so much more than a drawing of a face with a sealed-off mouth labelled with a street sign symbol and lettering, 'No Entry'. Which could have been, but I like to think not, "No access for therapist", but even here in the picture the black tight lip is doing more than indicating "no entry"; it can be a tight-lipped, "I will not speak out." Obviously there are almost limitless possibilities, here and throughout the rest of the picture. It is even possible that the red mouth area contains a sensual or sexual ingredient.

Usually I do not stay too long with these considerations because they can be something of a trap, though perhaps not intended to be, pulling the therapist away, too soon, from other possibilities. Certainly the mysterious mouth seems to be approached by the banana, the sharp fish and the unattractive apple. Although I do not feel that it is intended, this apple is so deadly-looking that my mind flashes back to the poisoned apple that is given to Snow White by her step-mother witch! Now we see that the imagination of the therapist is both a strength and a weakness!'

Thinking of this first session after many years have passed by and considering the painting, its production and what might have happened in the session, it is clear to me that the most important occurrence was the communication from the girl's sub-conscious to her conscious as she produced and perceived the picture. The best therapy would be from that process. Perhaps the most powerful expressions made were the black eye holes and the razor sharp eyebrows and nose lines.

While not wishing to describe here the long, complex and ultimately successful process of therapy over nearly a year, the girl spending time with separate weekly one-hour sessions with a psychiatrist and myself, I do need to indicate the good outcome.

The girl's expressive paintings became more and more abstract, with bold and increasingly bright colours. She shared increasingly more with the psychiatrist but told very little to me, the art therapist, treating me like a friendly fellow art enthusiast. Her art, however, I am sure gave her a satisfactory avenue of expression; "It loosens me up," she said. It was also, I think, a symbolic act, a sharing and even an approval of myself as a therapist, when she gave me the painting.

My colleague psychiatrist reported that the girl was clearly depressed by family stresses, in particular a very difficult relationship with her mother. There was never evidence of any abuse apart from a period of self-abuse when she would cut her arm, not severely, from time to time in the months preceding her clinic attendance. The cutting, happily, had come to an end for some reason, before her art therapy sessions began.

It did seem that the girl's difficulty was that of clinical depression within her early adolescence, which exaggerated the stresses that were in her family, especially the "love and hate relationship" – her words to the psychiatrist – with her mother. Her anorexia began with the rebellion of rejecting food that her mother prepared for her.

The outcome of her therapies was happily very successful: in retrospect the painting, 'No Entry', seemed to express a great deal of her sadness and anger. I believe that it may well have set her upon the road to recovery.

The following piece of writing from a different young lady who also had anorexia, while not telling us exactly how to treat those with this dangerous illness, does indicate what we should not do.

As to the question, "How should we use art therapy to help anorexics?" answers are proposed within many theories. Within my own work I have discovered that each client who comes my way is unique and what comes out at each session is therefore very individual, particularly perhaps with those suffering from eating disorders. I have found that my "Do as you wish," encouragement to troubled young people has proved successful because of the infinite possibilities of how he or she came to find themselves in this situation. Their case is unique.

The root of the problem is not supposed or necessarily exposed, in art therapy. The freedom of expression given to the client as in this case, perhaps while being also supported by another therapist working in a different mode, appears to give healing.

Helvi's Anorexia

Insights into the various attempts to treat a young person's anorexia, from an art therapy session with Helvi in Denmark

Halfway through a week in group therapy with myself, Helvi, a pleasant, slim but not too slim lady surprisingly presented me with the following. She said that I could make use of it in any way I wished. I circulated the document to many of my professional colleagues. I believe that it gives good advice.

'I felt so much shame… I was upset that people should know of my problem… When I was ill and thin they could see… then when I was fatter they referred to the change so I felt worse. It's so hard when people ask you about anorexia. You would feel so sensitive that your world would start to fall apart. There is shame. But you can feel strong because you have the power. The 'control' can be so bad for the family. The family must not let the anorexia take control.

'When I became bulimic there was so much shame, spending money and such. All your energy goes on the system… what to eat and what not to eat. It is then impossible to focus on the problem. I was a high achiever at skiing but realised I was not doing so well. That was a problem… I realised that I had to eat. I tried to eat non-fatty food. My parents realised and did not know what to do, immediately went into anger. Then the problem came. I had to eat (for example, eat before school…) Then I vomited and felt apathetic. It became worse from then.

'I did not know why it was happening and it would have been good if they had not gone to anger… if only they could have sat down to talk to me. I wanted to be cared for as I was. I was not satisfied with my achievements. I also had to keep on. The sport of skiing was all I seemed to be valued in. Without that I felt that I would be nothing. I did not like to hear things like, "You must get help… then you will quickly get back to skiing." I did not know why I had the illness. If my parents had worked hard with me to find the origin of the problem it would have been good.

'I met my first psychiatrist when I was eighteen years old. He just looked at me and made notes. I could sit for four hours and say nothing. I felt sure that he was trying to get me to be angry. I was determined not to be. It should be that the psychiatrist explains his approach and why he is meeting with the patient and discusses how this may or may not help. I cannot remember ever having such a discussion with a professional!

'Every person has his/her own individual way of eating. Force-feeding you fear most in your life. The "breakfast" situation should have been discussed. Not so much "Eat the breakfast!" It all started when I was fourteen years old. My older sister was okay. I had anger but we didn't argue in our house; that was why matters got worse. I now know that art therapy then would have helped me. I would have liked my parents to have seen that there were more sides to me than the sport/skiing success… it overshadowed every other aspect of me. I thought that it was the only thing that they cared about (but I guess it wasn't). It would have been so good for them to have said they loved me, loved me for what I am, not for what I was achieving or could achieve.

'When I was about twenty-seven or twenty-eight, I joined an Interest, or self-help, group for women with eating disorders run by women who have had such problems. No professionals – no outsiders. It was so good. It is about shame and hiding that shame. So much trying to explain, and then I met people who nod and say, "Oh, yes." They knew, so a lot of my shame went away. We went out to talk to nurses and doctors but I wasn't really well at that time.

'Once we went to talk to scientists and psychiatrists,

talking for fifteen minutes – it became two hours. It was okay but of course I was still unwell. I saw the great expert psychiatrist once a week for two years. The environment – desk, paper and volumes – he was always ten minutes late. Focussed on symptoms. Facts. Figures. Frequencies. Second time, I began the lies! He directed me week by week and I lied about the facts. Basically I thought, "Why see him if I can't be honest?"

'What would have been helpful would have been: a friendlier room – very important. He should not be writing all the time. He focussed too much on what was shameful to me. That was when the shame became worse... because I lied. He warned me of being also selfish, warned me of what might happen. He should have talked about evaluating the treatment – what did I think? I grew sick and tired of questions. It could have been good if the questions had been about the treatment. It would have been easier to be honest.

'It would have been good to have had the opportunity to see clinicians with different approaches, not to see lots but to have some flexibility. Psychodrama once a week for two hours helps me! I am the only one with a history of eating disorder but I can see that I have things in common with other people there. I have been in art therapy for six months. I have not thrown up since.

'I have always felt that I could not say that I am cured unless I had been symptom-free for two years. Now I feel sure that I will not fall back to anorexia. I have always had ups and downs. I don't try the "day-by-day" any more. I know that I am now normal. My mind is not thinking as it did, always about food... throwing up. Before, I could look in the mirror and think perhaps I might lose two kilos – it's always two, or two more and two more! Now I think that my life would have been much easier if I'd said, "Hello, Stupid, don't you have more important things to care about?" I realise that the two kilo thing is about something else. Then I have to consider that you cannot think of what's wrong in life when you're into anorexia/bulimia. It's just the food – you can't think about anything else.

'The psychodrama therapy, the role play, gives thoughts. At times you hear people saying your thoughts. The self-help group diminished my "shame". We learned, by the way, that therapy rules in the 'self-help group' are good!

'Art therapy helps me. It's difficult to describe how but for me it's very important to look at theory. I learnt that parts of my psyche were controlling me and I was not really controlling myself.'

It was very good of Helvi to actually ask me to make full use of these notes. I suppose that this was part of her 'sharing' and a wish to help others. I believe that most of all this clarification of her personal journey with words (even more clearly defined by the translation in her head into English) was very much part of her therapeutic process that week. Her comments should help therapists. She is an attractive woman in her late thirties but looks younger. Helvi's English is excellent and she is clearly a very intelligent and sensitive person. Her family are comfortably off and have several houses. To maintain confidentiality, I have altered some of the details in this narrative but the facts remain essentially unchanged.

I worked for a week with Helvi and fourteen others. My approach was, as with each individual, to encourage her within the group, working in the studio where she could 'share' alongside the other participants, to paint spontaneously and if possible to discuss the 'product' with me. As you can see from the above, she was very able at discussing her difficulties.

Certainly I felt that in the sessions Helvi came to understand aspects of herself better. There seemed to be a control theme in her three large and colourful paintings. Although abstract and in part beautiful and harmonious, there was a clear feeling of a balance between an unpleasant dark and 'edgy' grey area intruding onto an almost luminous orange-red area. In the last painting, the orange colour dominated. I felt that the grey pattern had something of a 'vampire' feeling, taking the energy from the rest of the painting.

It was clear that these large and colourful abstractions, encouraged by me but never with any directives from me, were an expression of Helvi's psychological state. On the paper there were dark shapes being balanced by energetic colours which I hoped indicated a triumph of good health over bad. I had a clear idea that this troubled young woman was giving her conscious self a better understanding of her difficulties and an optimistic 'view' of her potential for full healing. The art therapy was not cluttered by verbalisation, as other therapies had been for her.

Many theorists would understand the great value of a therapy which aims to help those suffering from anorexia by avoiding an emphasis on language. The acceptance and rejection of food begins, usually in a most natural way, in infancy. In our early days when we feed or are fed, our communication is not that of speech but of a multitude of actions including body and facial movements, babble, smiles, shouts, screams and eye contact or avoidance. Along with these are of course inner thoughts but not real inner language. This pre-language state is called somatic. Verbal description of 'feelings' is a sophisticated ability and while some of us manage well, others struggle and it is said the roots of anorexia connect with the somatic situation. It follows then that the anorexic may perhaps gain little from questioning, discussion and confrontation on the 'food issue'.

Expressive (or projective) therapy techniques may connect back to the somatic state. Art therapy should help. Whether it is avoidance of saying how she or he feels, or a genuine problem of thought, there is an opinion that people with anorexia find it particularly difficult to enter into 'talking therapy' for the reasons I have outlined here. Having no words for feeling is called the 'alexythymic state'; it seems that pictures can be discussed, if feelings cannot!

Before attending my sessions Helvi had attended many art therapy sessions with a female Danish therapist and she continued with these sessions after those she attended with my group. I would have liked to have had ongoing sessions with Helvi, because it seemed clear that she trusted me and I thought therefore, that I could help her to focus even better upon her paintings in a very positive way. Unfortunately, this could not be arranged and actually the change from a female therapist to a male therapist and back again was, Helvi told me later, a very positive happening for her.

One particular point made by Helvi was that a key word for her problem was 'shame'. Telling professionals of her problem focussed her shame. What a relief it must have been to discover psychodrama, the symbolical acting out with people she trusted of a problem and its origins, and art therapy, expressing and confronting feelings through paintings and connecting with them in a harmless way, where language and questioning were absent or minimal.

Chapter 12

Physical Disability and The Joy of Art

How can a person who has never been able to hold a brush or scribble a line begin as an artist? I no longer work specifically with physically and multi-handicapped children but have experience and writings from the past and thought that it might be useful to look back at my notes. Some of what follows includes jottings that I made around 1965 while working full time with disabled young people:

Let us consider a boy in a wheelchair who cannot hear, talk or walk; his hands are paralysed, he has little control above the waist and absolutely no control below the waist. He has learning difficulties. He has never painted or sculpted, perhaps rarely chosen what he would like to wear and although he can reject food as he is fed, there are no opportunities for choice even in feeding. If only this boy could paint, sculpt and draw, there would be opportunity for choice and experience of texture, form, colour and line. Why should he not have a chance to produce his own creative work? How should we approach such a disabled person?

Sit opposite and try to befriend him. He does not hear but he can see. Get some colourful paint and play with it, getting your fingers covered in paint, letting him see that this is fun. Wheel him up to a high table and sit next to him. Provide a paint dish and some nice paper. Stick your nose in the paint; bob your head and dot lots of spots over the sheet. Then put one of your very wet, messy fingers near to his nose. He does not seem afraid and the paint goes on. With any luck he copies you, bobs his head and makes some coloured dots. The pattern goes up on the wall. Applaud enthusiastically and put his name on the corner of the painting. He has made a start, smiling broadly. This is a true story; his name was Paul and he was nine years old.

Perhaps after you have shown how, he can bite from a piece of expanded polystyrene tile or packaging, creating a crude shape; naturally we have to take care here. He can then nose-paint this, or try with a brush held between his teeth. This will also go on display. He is now not only a painter, he is a sculptor. He has found some freedom. Access to special computerised equipment, especially computer graphic programs now give wonderful opportunities but when I began this work in the early Sixties there were no such things.

With Maria it was not the painted nose that was the major breakthrough, it was the big toe on her right foot. Richard typed pictures using a stick fastened to an elastic headband. Alec showed us how a chin can be used to roll and position strips of plasticine into shapes and figures. He would cut the pieces with his teeth, then assemble them with nose and chin. It is quite amazing to see the effect of such a permissive approach, especially when one comes across very handicapped young people who are given their first uninhibiting opportunity in art. Many go on to more difficult craft techniques and even machinery from such expressive beginnings. Confidence is gained and possibilities or unusual but effective physical controls are discovered.

When working for a period as a member of Care Staff, I came across Julie, a girl of nearly eighteen, who lived in an adult centre. She was physically handicapped, could not use her hands and propelled herself in her wheelchair by kicking with her left foot. She was unable to work in the centre workshop with all the other disabled people and was given 'drugs for depression'. Together we tried painting with brushes held between our toes. I was only marginally better than she was but she soon discovered that playing with paint was 'something to do'. We had fun. When I left her a week later I asked her to keep in touch. "Write me a postcard," I said. "Then I'll know how clever you've become with your toes." Three years later I was able to visit the centre and was deeply moved to see the same young lady at work. Julie was in the centre's workshop making woven rush seats on stools unaided, using only her feet. She greeted me warmly and said quite seriously, "I haven't sent you a post card because I can't write well enough yet."

Lorna was nearly 14, severely handicapped by cerebral palsy. She was still at her special residential school but was due to leave at 16. Totally dependent, Lorna had been loved and cared for and although delicate, she was in good health. She spent the day in her wheelchair, could not speak and apart from the odd smile or flutter of the eyelash, had never found a way to communicate clearly. It did not appear that she would be able to learn to read and was not even able to control her flailing limbs long enough even to point. Lorna was unsuccessful in all physical activities and the best she could do was, when in the right mood, grasp the paint rag just long enough to make a smudge on a large sheet of paper.

I showed Lorna my photograph of an equally handicapped but very bright young man using a paint stick on a headband. Would she like to try? A big smile indicated "Yes" and a headband was fixed to her head after she was shown the way in which it could be used. It became clear that she could not manage any control sitting in her wheelchair, so we tried her lying tummy down on a rubber wedge. In this position she managed to make windscreen wiper movements, which created some marks. Some staff were less than optimistic. A year later, she went to London to receive a special prize for her paintings from broadcaster Richard Baker, in conjunction with an exhibition produced by the Invalid Children's Aid Association.

While she was still at school, progress with her paintings led to Lorna being able to point with her head stick to a word board especially made for communication purposes, while sitting in her wheelchair. Through art she had learnt to communicate by written word. Visual concepts were already within her, awaiting expression. Sadly, in the past it was presumed that Lorna was of low intelligence. With a little help, she began her art work and moved fairly easily on, for the first time in her life, to communication with others. She became free of her prison.

I found as a young man, back in the late 1960s, that there were many amongst those who worked with the disabled who would tell you what not to do and a few who would tell you what to do. It might be, for instance, that a non-communicating child using his feet to make art-work should be discouraged from doing so in the view of some, because this unusual approach to overcoming one physical problem might lead to the child developing deformity in another part of his body. I battled this point once with a 'prohibiting' paediatrician and won.

I strongly believe that, while we must safeguard the handicapped, priorities must be established. Does the greatest need lie in physical maintenance, or in the expression of self? How limited life becomes if expression and communication are not seen as priorities. Every person should have the opportunity to make personal statements.

'Opportunity' is clearly the key word in working with people who have severe limitations. From the opportunity of being helped to discover that they can make marks they usually move on easily to make patterns and even pictures. If we need in these situations to see the 'psychological/therapeutic' aspect that comes from 'opportunity' we might perceive the process to be truly therapeutic through sheer joy, developing enthusiasm and improved self-respect and the confidence that goes with it.

I have seen that painting and sculpting assist special needs children in developing improved body controls and give emotional stability during and beyond that difficult adolescent period of their lives. In one residential school I was able to see wonderful progress over nine years. A similar effect is seen where children manage to improve physical control in a play situation when they had repeatedly failed to complete a similar task during physiotherapy.

Artistic Viewpoints

How we individually view art in general would be a component part of working with healing art. We find art assessed less and less from a purely "realistic" point of view, especially since the development of the camera and the rise in popularity of photography as a true form of art. History proves 'academic' judgement can be unjust and, with its rules of harmony and accurate representation, only one of the many valid approaches to art. Plotinus, a third century philosopher, proposed that "art should not merely be an imitation of material nature; it should be a point of departure of metaphysical experience, it should enable the spectator to come closer to the Divine Mind which has created them both, the subject and the evocation of the subject." The essence of this still applies.

In the diversity of work produced by artists today, whether amateur or professional, child or adult, we see many viewpoints and because of our exposure to various styles of art, we have a breadth of appreciation unknown in previous centuries. It is this that enables us to enjoy the varieties of artistic expression imposed or affected by disability. Adult primitive painting, resulting from a lack of artistic development, may be as enchanting as child art. Throughout history art has not improved but changed, maturing within the particular social context of attitudes.

Amongst the earliest known examples of representational painting are those in the caves of Lascaux in France. They are 17,000 years old and create an impression of realism through a suggestion of surface, form and sometimes movement, equal to any art that has followed. Humanity has only recently reached a point in time where we can be aware of art from many cultures past and present.

Nowadays we can appreciate many individual approaches; we may see them similarly effective in other places and times. It can be seen that symbolic device may, at one time, satisfy all aesthetic needs. While in another time other forms of description may be sought and if not found, the work is considered unsatisfactory. Thus one age or culture often has difficulty in understanding the priorities of another; for example members of isolated tribes may instantly recognise a familiar three-dimensional figure but if their culture's art is decorative and abstract instead of figuratively representational, they will not recognise a drawing of the same figure because it has only two dimensions. Our own culture in the West exposes us to examples of two-dimensional representation of form from infancy. Environment affects people's understanding of art. Cultures that have not felt a need to create a suggestion of depth are able instead to concentrate on perfection of design and decoration in two dimensions, as in Europe in the Middle Ages.

Perspective is the diminishing effect of distance creating apparent shrinkage and foreshortening. Today most children will eventually tackle theses problems of space in their pictures but if they do not naturally develop in that direction, it is wrong to force them. An adult, for instance, will see railway lines appearing to grow closer together as they move away, until they meet on the horizon. This is how he will draw it and his approach we call "objective". A child seeing the lines, will draw them parallel, which can be wrongly interpreted as "seen from above". The railway lines are not drawn to meet because the child, even while seeing that they appear to, knows they do not. This is "subjective" art. Which is the correct approach?

Another example of subjective art is seen in 'hieretical proportion', which has been used in many styles. In this, the more important the person is, the larger he is drawn, as in Ancient Egyptian art. Similarly, important parts of the body may be emphasised. I have seen definite exaggeration of shoulders on drawings by those who use crutches but distortion can usually be blamed on visual difficulties or problems of hand control.

With all these elements in mind, we may see the relevance of influences upon our own concepts when reacting to the art of special children.

The sketchy line and vigorous brushwork seen in the paintings by children tremulously affected by athatosis and ataxia has, in this day and age, particular fascination and success. It is only in the past century or so that we have been conditioned to see the vibrant quality in such efforts. Thanks mainly to the popularisation of the drawings and paintings of the French Impressionist painters and then later the Abstract Expressionists. We interpret the work as we uncontrollably let our minds fill the gaps and add to the information supplied. In this way incidentally, even the paralysed are creatively involved as they interpret an artist's work. We are attracted to and held by the paintings as our imagination is stimulated by them. If the images were much clearer, the qualities, particularly the suggestion of atmosphere, would be lost. Many other characteristics or artwork from special children gives special interest. Compelling effects can be seen in the distorted work of those with visual difficulties and those isolated by their handicap. Psychological disturbance itself can produce extremely sensitive and impressive creativity. Well-known examples could include the works of Van Gogh, Munch, Soutine and several current exhibitors but happily, it is not possible to be certain!

Artwork, therefore, may have special qualities when the mind or body of the artist is 'special'. Disabled artists usually have to put a very great deal of effort, energy, concentration and patience into their work. When we realise this, we may be tempted to lower our standards unduly. Ultimately there is no kindness in such discrimination.

Beginnings

It is a common misinterpretation that the artist's role is that of a communicator of ideas and images to others. I believe that the basic function of imaginative creativity is to communicate with oneself. The most lasting expressive work has been created primarily from a desire to satisfy the severest of all critics – the artist himself and these creations have rarely harmonised with the current trends. Where is the value in coaxing a child to make pictures determined by ourselves? There is no real boost to self-esteem and the adult-led end product might have a sophistication that would confuse the child.

The old concept of language development was that when speech is available, the child can express his or her inner thoughts. Now we know that the early sounds and attempts to copy feed back and stimulate the advancement of thought. The spoken word and the inner language make for intellectual development. It is not generally understood that similar things can happen with concept of line, form and colour. As the child manipulates with finger or toe and if he clearly sees results in puddles of colour and crude scribble, his concepts advance enabling him to further develop graphic symbolism. If children with learning difficulties produce scribbles of paint and heaps of rubbish glued to a board that do not conform to our own aesthetic ideals of 'pictures' and 'models', remember that they may well be developmentally important to them.

It seems to me that when children are involved in the creative process, however primitive, the result, if really from them, is remembered. Unlike much of their class work, there is more chance of retention and meaning because a: the processes gone through are necessarily within the child's present ability and b: the resulting concrete success becomes a meaningful internal as well as external image. As a developing personality repeatedly externalises an internal idea or creates a partly accidental scribble that is completely their own, they accept a new image to progress from. The emergence of an expression becomes, if perceived by the creator, surely a unique and personal stepping stone to the next stage of development.

So it is that seemingly meaningless creations which have little value to us can have developmental value for the child; a very interesting topic covered later in this book.

Ideally the helpful grown-up should encourage the child to invent and express ideas with a wide range of play materials, in a friendly and relaxed atmosphere, ensuring that opportunity is given to investigate colours, textures and shapes. At times during these activities the child should if possible be allowed to see other children at play. Play and art activities can give more positive stimulation where there is group involvement. When the child has special needs, the stimulus often needs to be stronger and the encouragement greater, gently encouraging but never dictating. It is especially important to let the child decide what to do and how he should attempt it. In art activity special needs children may just need extra stimulation and success – and therefore increased confidence – not often found by them elsewhere.

I believe then that joyful expressive activity can involve, exercise and perhaps in some cases, give therapy by helping to improve confidence, body control and general development.

The beginnings of art, the scribble and daub, are play motivated. As a child can express little without experience we have to ensure that he has opportunities to involve himself with sensations and has available objects and boxes of things, if possible collected by the child himself, that will give tactile experience. Such games as smearing the table top with wet soapy hands and finger painting large pebbles are examples of good beginnings in art-play.

Achievement is essential to show the child that, whatever his disability, he can make some sort of mark on his own. We may assist him when necessary but his body must be involved. The first work of his that he sees displayed on the wall might be a toe print, nose print, wheelchair mark, or perhaps a form bitten out of expanded polystyrene. What is essential is the uninhibiting influence of the adult.

Special Problems

Often those who have begun art using foot, mouth or headband find it difficult to move on from their rigid markings, such as short jabs and crosses, to the cursive and round shapes that wrist movements easily allow. With a free approach, the artist may be encouraged to move on to simple tree or lollipop shapes. If the foot movement makes the tree ill-formed in the attempt to create curves, it will still satisfy. Similar distortion in a face may inhibit further attempts, but trees and hills are friendly. Vertical and horizontal control can be encouraged by moving your finger over the paper, daring the artist to paint your finger nail.

Modified equipment should not be given to those who can manage with the normal – it can happen! Large plastic, heavy-bottomed bowls with large brushes are useful, as are 'G' clamps and bench hooks for steadying works for those with spasms. With scraper boards, where a layer of ink is scratched from a white ground to reveal the white, as well as the proper sharp tools a stick with a knob of glass paper can produce fuzzy shapes. Large crayons and fibre pens are effective and ball-point and gel pens may sometimes suit; there should be many choices. One youth with uncontrollable athoid shaking who was particularly interested in lino cutting never cut himself, although the tools he used were normal.

Some say that they do not like to paint because it is messy. This often indicates that they make a mess with the paints and that the mess embarrasses them. The only thing to do is to remove the embarrassment by showing how to enjoy making a colourful mess. To un-inhibit adults and children, once they have been inhibited, is the most difficult problem. Viewing exhibitions of modern art may assure the children of the 'respectability' of such 'messy' paintings. It's always a great idea to visit art galleries.

Structures made of junk embedded in clay, putty or plaster can be a good introduction to three-dimensional works. Also particularly useful are impressions in plasticine made with fingers, elbows or the application of various round forms. Into these impressions plaster may be poured and when the plasticine is removed, a plaque with raised forms results. Rags slipped into wet plaster, which is easily tinted with powder colour, and pushed onto a board can have extra paint added when it sets. In this way a pleasant abstract relief can be made – messy but effective.

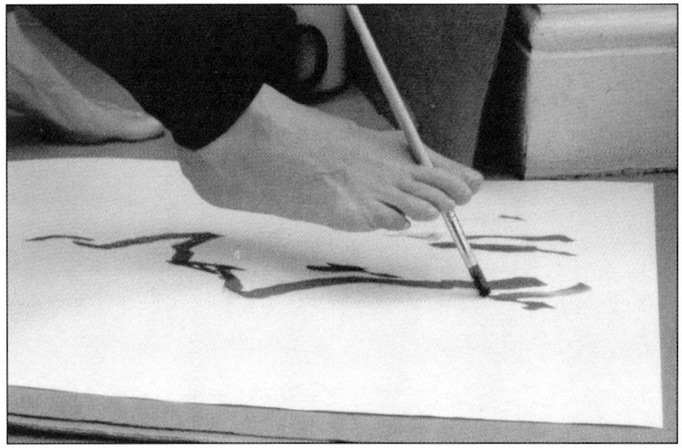

Kitchen foil interestingly accepts impressions of forms such as keys and coins and it may be pushed against, folded around and pressed into the forms of the body, especially hands and arms. This will reveal, when pulled away, the basic form which can be immediately hung from the wall.

When the artist holds the brush with his teeth or uses a headband, the brushes need to be the unvarnished type and the table and chair at exactly the practical height, not too difficult to organise. Those using their toes should be comfortably seated, brushes or pencils being placed in a short jar and/or a bowl made of a material other than glass, which is on the floor. The paper may be pinned to the floor or onto a board upon the floor. The board itself may have to slope. Techniques and materials must vary but with older children if skills have been discovered and enjoyed, I can see no point in constantly changing.

It can be important for young people to be stimulated by works done by others around them. They will often wish to try something that an older child is doing and it is often good to let them try. The developmental movement the child makes over the years in art will be from exploration, involvement and observation to controlled work with colour, tone, line and shape and form. This would ideally include 'additive' – for example, clay models – and 'subtractive' – for example, carving – three-dimensional works and an understanding of what printing means; potato prints may be a good start. Encouragement should not consist solely of praise; the works will always be "interesting" but rarely "excellent". Critical comment will enhance the effect of praise at another time.

It is important to be sure that the child knows how much help he is getting. One severely physically handicapped boy told me when we first met, "I have just had a painting hung in an exhibition. Dad always helps me and he's very good at art." This lad so quickly developed skills holding the paintbrush between his teeth, it is sad to reflect that his father, who did all the painting while his son watched and advised, thought that his method was the best way to help the boy, when in fact he was gaining little from the experience.

If art is treated as fun but with independence considered a priority, all should be well. Any failures, and failures can be educational, must be followed by a successful activity. For example, if a child was unsuccessful in an attempt at drawing, it could be followed by an experiment with accidental paint effects. We could puddle colour onto a smooth surface and onto this drop paper, thereby achieving crude 'prints'. The best of the resulting 'prints' could be selected by the child and used in some decorative way, perhaps simply glued upon a large sheet of paper. This will give a positive result, whereas the drawing did not.

If the child sees that artistic freedom is allowed, he will try – and should be allowed – to be destructive, creative, or simply very messy, whatever the moment demands. Destruction can be a good introduction to sculpting in soft soap, plasticine and polystyrene blocks. Hammers, some with sharpened ends, fairly blunt chisels, rasps, files and blunt-ended round knives with large handles are useful. Naturally we need to make sure the young person is safely supervised. Some who show difficulty with tools may have the handles

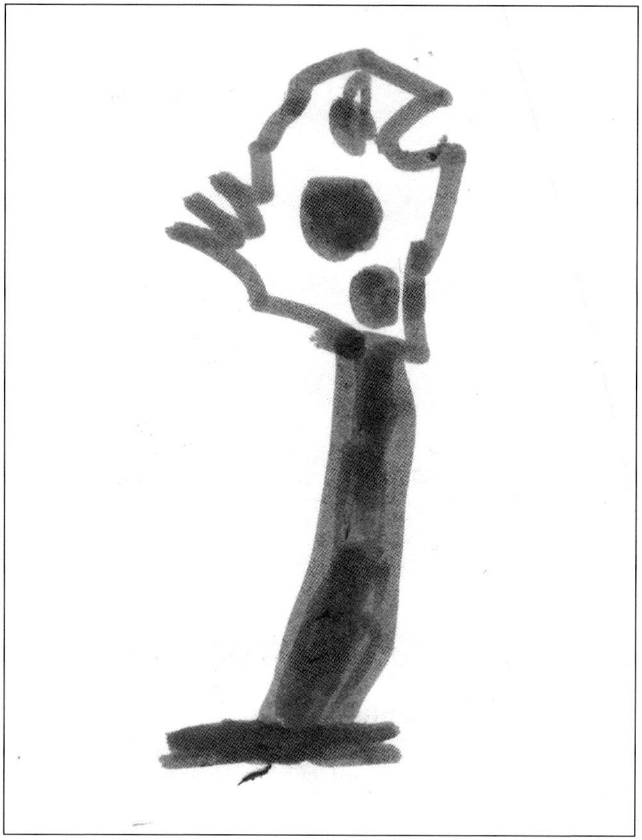

padded and it is also useful to have plenty of flattish, blunt-edged weights around, such as stones and lead blocks, to steady materials for those with unsteady hands. It needs to be said that some young artists I worked with had been told that their 'less able' hand or limb was 'bad', while the other was 'good'. This is so negative. There should be a 'clever' hand and a 'less clever' hand. Enough problems exist without the idea that the body has 'bad' bits!

Three-Dimensional Work

We learn that proper interpretation of two dimensions must be preceded by an understanding of three dimensions. It is wrong to suppose that every child progresses to abilities with three-dimensional work after achieving drawing controls. Where learning problems exist I feel that it can be advantageous to try carving simple shapes, as this is a stimulating experience. The limitations of the sculpting media may be, in some cases, a positive thing and less frustrating than too easily yielding clay. The beneficial effect on hand function of play with modelling clay is easily understood but it is often overlooked that a child who cannot draw or work well with clay and plasticine may be able to carve!

I know of one very unsteady young lady who could cope with a rasp, holding it with both palms pressed tightly together against the handle, carving deep patterns into a soft stone block. She was never happy working with plasticine and clay because of her 'palm-down' hand reflex pattern (a problem which because of her disability could never go away: she was unable to perform pincer movements with her fingers) made it extremely difficult to bind the pieces together.

On one occasion, a boy in a wheelchair who could not use his feet or hands and managed only poor work with the brush held unsteadily between his teeth, asked to sculpt. For years he had managed little and turned to a rather passive physical existence, until one day he saw one of our girls who had no useful hand function happily making grooves in soft stone by pushing a rasp, flat upon the block, with her plimsoll feet. A block of this synthetic stone was set in a vice upon a bench at his knee level and a large-handled rasp was put into his palm while his fingers were pressed around it. This was, in a few seconds, dropped but we persevered. Each time the rasp clattered to the floor, the boy and the other members of the group laughed.

We tried with the rasp placed into the right hand as it rested on the boy's lap. The left hand swung over, eventually joining the other hand in a semblance of gripping. Gradually the tool swung outwards but the movement was, with the weight, less erratic. As the tool bumped down on the surface of the stone it came almost to rest, his hands between his knees. Using the friction as an aid, the boy adjusting the placing of the rasp over to the required place; as the tool bit into the surface a proper rhythm replaced the wobble as his body moved to and fro. A channel was soon cut into the block this way. The movement available was unsuitable for drawing or painting but with this technique a design was eventually produced. He had for the first time, at the age of 12, made something with his hands. The only aids given were the placing and turning of the stone in the vice and, once or twice each session, replacing the rasp onto his lap.

When faced with chisel, rasp and files the basic technique is seen to be a process of subtraction. The removal of form from a rectangular block tends to create geometric shapes. With the crude figure carvings for instance, the legs may easily be straight and of an equal length, while shoulders and facial features can have an easy symmetry. The great difference is that a drawing starts only when the mark is applied to the paper and 'irregularities' are common, while a carving begins with the basic block form and while the work progresses, continues to relate to that form. With modelling this does not apply, but where a stick figure is produced from crossed ropes of modelling material, there is more possibility for some of producing symmetry so difficult to achieve in drawing. It is perhaps surprising that for some a piece of soft stone, or breeze block, is more user friendly than clay or paint!

Back in the early seventies I sensed that some special needs children had depressive forces affecting, and sometimes damming, artistic expression and communication. I know of one particular case where within a year or so, a form of artistic expression, through a beginning of an interest in painting, was seen to kindle, or perhaps rekindle, his zest for life. In this case a glum boy came for the first time to my art class and after much hesitation drew a few watery unlinked lines and followed this by mixing some powder paint in a palette. It was obvious he enjoyed washing his brush more than painting on paper! By the end of the session he had produced only a few lines and at the last moment obliterated even these.

I tried to encourage the boy but he was suspicious and reluctant to paint, wanting only to talk. Whenever it was possible, we did so. I continued to place paper and paints before him and as I assisted others, he would doodle with lines of muddied colour. More and more of his chattering turned to his surprising view that, although in fact he was cerebrally palsied, he denied any connection with "those spastics" and was, he said, "normal but not yet walking". As the weeks went by the boy, not considered by the school's psychologist to be disturbed in any way, confided more and more in me. While he said he was never allowed out of the school to meet non-spastics, in reality he would refuse to go out even when transport was supplied. One day he ceased his abstracts of dull lines and produced without any directive, an easily distinguishable, violently erupting volcano. From that time on his paintings were entirely different and colourful. He created an almost unending stream of pictures and patterns, never needing direction, and expressed a great enthusiasm for art. The boy did, unfortunately, continue with some of his odd comments but generally – and staff remarked on this – was a very much happier person (and an art enthusiast). This young man, and others I was to meet, led me eventually into art psychotherapy, where I was to come across many angry volcanoes.

Three young people who gained much from their time in the artroom

Let us look back into my personal notes made around the late Sixties and early Seventies, when I was a full-time art teacher at a residential special school. Most of the children were very physically handicapped and it was wonderful to see the joy that they found in discovering that they could, despite all their difficulties, be 'real artists' and even for one very disabled teenager, "a real artist and a real person". What follows is gleaned from what I learnt – and I think the teacher will always learn very much from those he is teaching! – plus some reflections I made at that time.

ROBERT: At nearly seventeen, he is extremely keen on reading, writing, music and painting. He is well liked for his pleasant sense of humour and, although he is rather weak at spelling, copes well with education. His burning ambition is to have his writing published and make a living as an author.

Robert, strapped in a wheelchair, has little control of movement and no speech. He was born, after a long and difficult labour, with his umbilical cord wound twice around his neck and did not breathe after it was loosened for fifteen minutes. At first it seemed that all would be well but after six months it was seen that he was not developing naturally and was making uncontrollable reflex responses seen only in the newborn. These he still makes.

At eight months he was taken to Great Ormond Street Hospital for Sick Children where it was decided that his asphyxiation at birth had damaged his brain, causing severe athetoid cerebral palsy. It was doubtful that he would ever walk, talk, move his limbs properly or have good intelligence. At two and a half years, Robert attended the Bobath Clinic in London where, for two years, he received intensive physiotherapy. Next he moved to the first of the five schools he was to attend over the following fourteen years. He has never learnt to sit, stand, crawl, feed, toilet or dress himself but propels his wheelchair by kicking at the ground with his right foot.

To communicate with others he must wear a rod fixed to a headstrap, which he taps onto an alphabet board that always hangs from the back of his wheelchair. With this same unicorn-like headpiece or 'beak' he has learnt to type and, when a pencil or brush is fixed to its end, draw and paint. Not surprisingly, his favourite school subjects are English and Art. He has tried unsuccessfully to speak using a mechanism for amplifying sounds in the larynx and a specially adapted electric wheelchair. To stop his arms waving wildly about, he has both strapped to the arms of his wheelchair.

Though affected by athetoid spasms, Robert's paintings show a very good understanding of natural colour, shape and proportion. He admits to brief periods of depression, though I have never seen any reflection of this in his warm and often very expressive pictures. His writings reveal a part of his personality not evident in his pictures, a glimpse of innermost thoughts and frustrations. Incredibly, his intelligent mind appears only slightly affected by his imprisoning, cruel handicap. Does he fully realise his limitations? His life has always been a sheltered one, with assistance always at hand. A poem by Robert seems to indicate new feelings of sexuality and what he calls "terrifying reality":

'Through death, life, a spectrum of colour
I followed the butterfly love
Through black death,
The green, orange, purple, red, brown, grey of life.
Not missing a single flick of its wings,
Until, whispering in the wind, reality confronted me.
No McCartney song about happy love,
No poem by Wordsworth,
Instead of romance – sex.
Instead of running through grass fields –
Beds, beds, beds.
Harsh, terrifying reality.
I could not bear it.
It came through the one crack in my protective shell –
The crack the butterfly of love made.'

Robert's painting shows little or no poetic symbolism; it is as if he projects his most personal imagery through his more competent technique of typing while in his paintings he contents himself with struggling to define more clearly shape and form.

As far as naturalistic painting is concerned, he has two difficulties: (i) poor brush control due to the limitations imposed by his 'beak' and (ii) every developing artist's problem of portrayal of form which depends on accurate observation and memory.

Robert's paintings show vigorous brushwork and inaccuracies evident are not so unusual. They are simply a less than perfect understanding of the subtleties of shaping and placing. Like most people, he tends to over-simplify and bring the shapes towards a more geometric form. With his inevitable shaky athetoid brushmarks, the larger the painting the more detailed it may appear and the vibrant impressionist manner gives a special quality and no limitation is apparent.

Robert's painting is not faulted so much by poor control as by his insufficiently critical vision. When asked whether a particular group of angles are correct he will more often than not indicate his mistakes and correct them.

As Robert cannot speak of his artistic pursuits, he has typed the following for me:

'Art I use in a general way for anything creative, whether paint, wax, ink or thoughts. Drawing, essay, poem or imagination, they are all art to me. I cannot remember when I started painting, it was in the far distant past

when I was about four years old. At first I painted with my left foot, nothing much – mostly big mix-ups. I wasn't very steady or particularly artistic. Then when I was about nine or ten I had my "beak". It took me at least a year for me to become so-so-okay, but two years to get proficient.

'Painting to me is an opposite to boredom but it can become boring. I sometimes "paint" pictures in my mind which I want to paint, but I don't very often find that I am capable of painting it.'

In my experience as a painter and observer of painters I discount the often-heard idea that a person knows and has a clear vision in his mind of the picture he wishes to create but has not the skill to portray it in a graphic way. I believe instead that the imagined picture has a similar quality to those parts of dreams where we can accept the particular concept of a person or thing, without being aware of its appearance in detail. It is that the idea is vague, I think, and cannot be properly defined. It is not a problem of lack of skill.

Robert might, for example, need an oak tree in one corner of his picture but in his imagination 'oak tree' is little more than a poorly defined symbol which cannot be observed and copied effectively. As experienced artists can construct a realistic tree from singular and composite memories of other trees and parts of trees, carefully observed and perhaps drawn in the past, it is not that Robert's skill in reproducing his mind pictures is poor, it is that these pictures are lacking as yet in information and ill-defined conceptually. The present weakness in his paintings would not appear to stem from his handicap as his vigorous technique imposed by his athetoid condition has no weakening effect if the picture is large enough. In illustrative work he needs to observe more carefully and review and criticise his drawings as he progresses. With imaginative work the handicap is insufficient knowledge of natural configuration. These are in fact normal and common faults in all aspiring painters.

Robert, suspicious of praise, enjoys constructive criticism and dislikes the attitude that leads people to say that his paintings are good merely because of his physical disability. He and many others similarly affected have assured me that this approach to their work is prevalent even amongst parents and close friends.

In the art room Robert will, more usually than not decide what he wants to do. He always mixes his own colours and attempts a variety of subjects. Even if he somehow learnt to speak, Robert has indicated that he thinks that he would not like a helper to interpret his instructions onto paper in art, as is perhaps done in some special schools and centres. Once he is prepared to begin, he decides for himself and does as he wishes without having to ask for further assistance, as he must for most of his occupations. With painting he can practise that very individual activity of choosing.

It is perhaps surprising that such a severely affected person can have apparently unimpaired visual perception. Tactile experience in such a child is very limited but he readily perceives and translates his vision in a graphic manner. If a 'normal' artist wanted to depict, for instance, an area of carpet, he or she conceives qualities of shape, colour and tone and automatically relates to memories of sensation, especially touch, relating to similarly textured fabrics. As he does he mentally feels. The artist and sculptor Henry Moore has talked of the artist's perceptual problem of "comprehending form in its full spatial existence" and the continued striving "to get the solid shape, as it were, inside his head". It is an enigma that Robert and others who have never really held anything appear to be able to do this.

As yet Robert has not really sculpted but he has impressed crude marks approximating figures, on clay, so they appear in the negative. I have poured plaster upon the clay and later when the plaster was set, torn the clay off to reveal the forms created by those impressions.

As I mentioned previously it is no use excluding an activity just because it appears that a child cannot cope; better to let them try and if they cannot manage introduce an aid and later withdraw it if it is at all possible to do so. If in the end the task proves to be too much, then they have learnt something of their limitations and we must next give them a simpler task that we know they can manage.

The most must be made of Robert's drive and determination and all avenues of expression must be explored, offering him opportunity to experiment and practise.

Soon he will leave school and his only independent function will be that of writer/artist.

(Robert went on to have his poems published in books and magazines but I lost touch with him.)

ANDREW: Unlike Robert, Andrew has no need of a wheelchair. He is cerebrally palsied and affected in his legs, though he moves well with two sticks. Nearly seventeen, Andrew is nearing the end of his grammar school education and will soon be looking for work. His favourite subject is English and his favourite hobby swimming.

Andrew has two brothers and two sisters who are perfectly able. He was premature and one of twins; his brother died at seven days old. No abnormalities were noticed in the remaining child until he was nine months old, when it was seen that he could not yet lift his head and his legs were rather rigid. Soon after his second birthday, Andrew went to stay in a hospital where he had constant physiotherapy. During his almost three-year stay in the hospital he learnt to walk with some assistance and obtained a satisfactory education.

Andrew's parents, when he was five and a half, applied to the Spastics Society (now Scope) for a place for him at one of their residential schools. The assessment panel were impressed by his alert, talkative and friendly manner. At that time the educational psychologist found that the Stanford/Binet Intelligence Scale indicated a mental age of six years while Andrew was five years and eight months.

At present attending a special school, Andrew shows a lively interest in the arts. His appreciation and understanding is far in advance of his ability, as with many people. He loves to read but his writings are marred, but not stifled, by weak spelling. While it becomes more apparent his spelling may never be very good, his work is nevertheless considered to have real feeling, imagination and descriptive ability, compared with the rest of his class.

Andrew writes (I have not corrected his slight mis-spellings):
'One can walk at any time through the Coltswolds and see many beauties of nature. The best time I think is Auteumn, at this time of year the leaves of the trees start to change coler and if you walke through a copes in the early Auteumn just before sunset you would see a paradise of all the coler and splener of nature. There would be great trunks still bending under the weight of Summer foliage. Only this canopy would be a profusion of multicoloured reds, browns and yellows, added to this the suns rays would shooe through the leaved giving the green moss at almost blue appearance and all this would send an optical haze of coolers before your eyes.
'... On a cold auteumn night some leaves will be tossed and blown so far and high they will reach once again the very hight they fell from.'

He is displeased with his spelling and handwriting but thinks the latter will not improve because his hands, he thinks, are rather clumsy. Andrew will soon be sitting G.C.E. exams and as yet he has no idea what he will do when he leaves school, but I am sure that he will not have great difficulty in finding some sort of work. He is sensible and sociable.

Andrew is intrigued by his 'strange way of drawing'. Five years ago in psychological testing, he was seen to have 'visual perceptual and visual motor difficulties', having some confusion in understanding what he sees and problems with eye-hand co-ordination. He has difficulties with his eye/motor co-ordination, resulting in poor drawing control, and poor understanding and recognition of shape and symmetry. I have seen Andrew improve much with repeated attempts; because of his love of art, he perseveres and achieves. I think that it would be a different matter, and less effective therapeutically, if he were given specific eye-hand training programmes by his occupational therapist. It is a matter of Andrew trying again and again, aiming to portray ideas in pictures, rather than attempting special exercises. He has learnt to look more carefully and to do his very best to control pencil, pen and brush. Though he has these visual difficulties, he now does better than we would expect.

In the art room, over two years he has discovered that he is able to improve his simple but charming drawings. His attempts have shown him that despite his problems, with enthusiasm and hard work better skills can be learnt. Interestingly as his art became more mature, though still in some ways naïve, he became more confident with his writing and spelling.

DIANA: A charming sixteen year old nearing the end of her secondary school education, Diana's main interest is fashion and her favourite school subjects are needlework, art and typing. She has, as yet, no idea what she will do when she leaves school and is aware of increasing interest in all things romantic. Though she has physical problems including a slight speech defect and an unsteady gait, her outlook is, happily, normal.

Diana writes:

'Someone,
Someone to wait for
every night at eight
someone to overcome
when all my fears are near.
Someone to comfort me when I'm sad,
someone to love me when I'm in love
someone to walk with me every Sunday
someone to say good morning makes my day
Four o'clock, a walk round the block
Oh, will I never meet that somebody
Well, like you?

I include Diana's poem, not as a romantic decoration but to show that through her typewritten work, she manages to express, without any real embarrassment, her personal feelings. This, I am sure, is a most important contributory factor in her general emotional stability. When she first came at the age of twelve to the residential school, she was very emotional, easily upset and homesick, very much a little girl lost.

Her handwriting is so unsteady as to necessitate constant practice with the typewriter and she has over the years, improved remarkably at it. She has some difficulty with her speech and uncontrollable facial movements which embarrass her but with her typing, unlike her distorted handwriting, she can write and communicate well and on an even standing with most.

Diana has been affected by cerebral palsy since birth, especially on her right side. Her speech difficulty stems from her poor muscular co-ordination, which results in immature-sounding and apparently undeveloped articulation (dyslalia). She had had regular speech therapy for thirteen years and, when viewing her involuntary facial movements, it is remarkable how well she does speak. Diana is one of those happier cases where, since her infancy, she has had good therapeutic treatment from speech and physiotherapists. She now manages very well.

Brush and paint are friendlier to a child than a pen and Diana is always very happy and relaxed when painting, never showing frustration. Perhaps this is because she is never over-ambitious. Art for her is a pleasant period of recreation, simple fun, and there is none of that determination and urgency seen in Robert's and sometimes Andrew's work. Her speech disability has now become quite mild and many of her personal qualities are reflected in her naïve but charming pictures. She tells me that art is "so relaxing".

Here I have to point out that the simple joy of making art is in itself cheering and therapeutic in a simple and very natural way. The act of creation satisfies and the physically limited can, in a very personal way, give vent to pent-up emotions through the process of this creativity. This is an especially important consideration when dealing with those who have difficulty with communication.

Confidence and an awareness of self identity can come from artistic development. How this confidence can help generally has to be seen to be believed.

There are many special needs people who need constant supervision, directions and assistance with everything that they do, often with the exception of drawing, painting and typing. It is vital that they should develop their skills so that they may have at least one individual satisfying and perhaps independent role to play in adult society. Most 'normal' children will eventually turn away from forms of pictorial expression, whereas others with fewer expressive outlets may involve themselves more and more with artistic activities. It is of paramount importance that these young people have every chance to do so.

A Crucifixion

Barry made a very modern model of the 'crucifixion' in the art room without any help (see next page). It took him about twenty minutes to produce. I was busy assisting eleven other severely disabled twelve year olds. Barry exclaimed with a look of exaltations upon his face "I did that... didn't know I could!"

I had given Barry a little board and pieces of plasticine at his request and had left him to it. Barry having no hand control whatsoever and sitting in a wheelchair managed to position the board on the raised table top using his chin and his nose. He had then rolled, and once or twice bitten the plasticine in to lengths. After positioning chosen pieces onto the board with his nose and chin Barry had pressed very hard upon the pieces so that they stuck to the board, making the form of a crucifixion. "Has that made your day?" I asked Barry. He excitedly answered, "Made my day! More like it's made my year!" In the months that followed Barry became an ever increasingly enthusiastic mouth painter, managing very well with a brush between his teeth.

I have in my possession one of the plaster casts copies of Barry's 'crucifixion' and from time to time I reflect on how this stylised sculpture may reflect the artists periodic painful times from the surgery that attempted to improve his physical situation. But most of all I appreciate its artistry and remember the joy that it brought Barry. The most important aspect must surely be that this subject was chosen and created independently without help or direction from others. This is Barry's own personal expression with a mixture of suffering and joy.

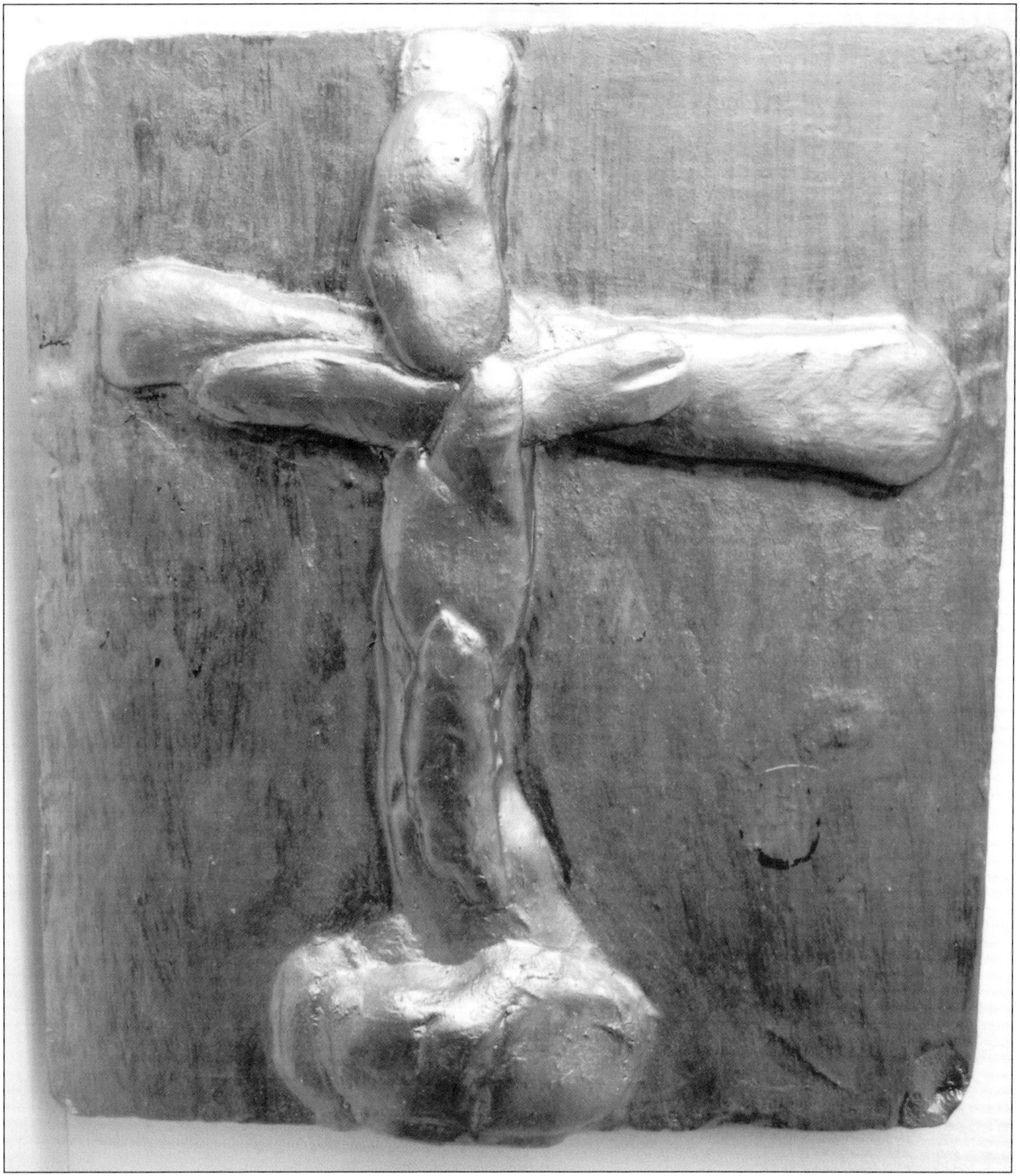

By Barry, using his nose, chin and teeth

Chapter 13

Pictures from Young Minds

My university research indicated several avenues of development in children's mark making, not just from marks to pictures as seemed evident in my research in the Seventies. A simple dot or line may represent a person or action. Children do produce a much wider repertoire of mark making than most adults are aware of, especially 'assemblies' and 'named' markings which are not seen by observers as descriptive. Representational marking, not picturing begins at around two years. Crude 'face' is discovered but is not of great interest at that time. The child has yet to learn that this type of marking is what society requires. Some sort of marking which holds a meaning within a completely individual and private process develops and continues to develop, I believe, as the 'picture making' (representational) ability develops, although it is not as easily seen and understood by onlookers. This was a new discovery made within the university but I have not until now published any of the findings.

Early marking should be seen as the evidence of a behaviour, the movement of the child and something that can be influential to that child's development as he or she considers what is occurring in time and space as the marks extend. The art-product, unlike the rest of the behaviour, remains and may well be briefly considered by the perceiving child as evidence of 'self'. A simple mark or line can, it seems, represent all or part of self, others, experiences, things and, perhaps, almost anything. These certainly at a very early stage become for the child 'representational', but to the adult just scribbled or abstract markings. What is easily seen as representational or realistic marking has come to be called 'drawing' or even 'figurative drawing' by adults. This is misleading, as the 'non-figurative markings' may be for the young creator, 'representational'!

It is likely, I think, that a curve, near-closure or enclosure may extend the idea of the brief mark as relevant to 'self'. The new suggestions of shape show the possibility of edge and a sign which has an inside and an outside. Certainly the idea of marking within an enclosure is surprisingly present before the child's first birthday. The enclosure sign, it seems, gives a strong idea of a container whether it be house, home, shop, person, self or object, but quite a different form from the first non-figurative but representational-to-the-child marks. This is a 'container shape' but not necessarily a body shape.

The infant's line, at least at eighteen months, generally represents, or seems to represent, movement, although it later comes to mean 'edge of' rather than self, person, object or happening.

It was very important within my study to mention those concepts referred to as 'subjective' and 'objective'. Infant art is generally subjective but there are surprising possible exceptions which seem, when observed, to suggest a view of lateral, as opposed to the usual – and adult – logical-vertical, thought process and development in the child. All so very complicated! While it may be seen that even at three years the child might copy, in an objective way, a toy or familiar three-dimensional objects, it was apparent to me that there is a to-ing and fro-ing from one experimentation in line and shape to another. It seems that the child can move to and fro from objective to subjective, unlike most adults. This finding was contrary to previous research.

At the World Conference in Infant Psychiatry in Lugano, Switzerland with my colleague Dr Janeck Dubovski, I presented my research into the development of mark-making by infants. I had utilised multi-camera split screen filming as the children drew freely, recording attention and posture as well as the work of the young artists. The following month, I made a modified and practical presentation to art therapy students at Ulriksholme, Denmark. This was of great interest to my friend the psychologist Vibeke Skov, who suggested a sort of role-play or game for her art therapy students, to give a personal and easily remembered experience which might give an insight into what could really be occurring as infants made marks, to look more at the process, rather than the product. This would, of course, contrast greatly with our own adult personal idea of 'art'. While not really allowing us to perceive as an infant does, it makes us think twice about any urge to interpret markings in an adult way. I suggested types of play with paper and crayon and I led them about the room. According to the students my game of 'I'm an infant playing with marks' made them experience something like the following:

'Here is a piece of paper upon the floor and it is very, very attractive to me. I know that if I took a crayon and marked the paper I would change it. Now I have marked the paper. There is a little line of colour. The space around the mark is now already changed; although it is not a mark, it is a space around the mark but the mark makes all of the sheet rather different.

'Now I watch the crayon move. It is just as interesting as the line itself. I can feel time passing as the line moves. I can feel that the mark is showing my movements. It is fast, slow, wobbling or wavering. It is cutting up the blankness of the paper. Look how now the line makes a shape. Now it stops as I stop. It seemed to have a life of its own but it is me who gives it life. It stops and I feel okay. I am not really stopped.

'I start another line on a piece of paper and again I feel that time passes, the line gets longer. The line is part of me, part of my movement and shows me and reminds me of space and time.

'The next line I make starts near to me and I watch it move away from me. It seems to connect with me.

'An adult is coming to pick up my paper and, I think, is going to put it up on the wall where it should not be. It is an "on the floor" paper. She is looking for "up/down" shapes and even perhaps a picture.

'But here's another piece of paper, a bigger piece upon the table not the floor. I've got the blue crayon and I'm moving my mark across the paper. I'll go slow; now fast and trying skidding around the corners. The line will let me explore most of this paper. But my blue line is getting everywhere on this paper and it grows through space as well as through time. I am thinking that it could even go through the table onto the floor, but then I hold the crayon and the paper and I move with them through the air and we rush around the room until I drop the paper from the crayon. I don't want the paper and I'll soon forget it, but I play with the crayon for a little while. I have not, in fact, really looked at the marks upon the paper, I was only interested in where the line might go as my crayon moved and the only interested in my crayon.

'There is another piece of paper on the table. I will mark it, fold it, mark it again, unfold it, mark it again and turn it over to make lines on. But I'm not going to see what it all looks like, because with my other hand I've already dropped another piece of paper on the floor and I think I will play with that. (Grown-ups will ask me, "What are your pictures about?" so I will I suppose have to think of something to say.)

'This big piece of paper on the floor is nice. I am making big curves that cross over each other and I think about "things"! I have made interesting shapes.

Shape is different from line. I am thinking about shapes with somethings in them. Some shapes are Mummy I think but those two little dots are, I think, an ice cream and my grandmother... at least they are for the moment. There is a big squiggle, which is me and my tummy. There is an "outside" to the squiggle and an "inside". All these lines are very different from all my other lines that I have made today, so I will now do a roundy-round line to be Daddy and look! As I put marks in the 'roundy"-round" they become Daddy's eyes, mouth and nose. This is fun but nearly not as much fun as my other marks.'

The language recounting the experience is not, of course, that of an infant!

According to the students the exercise had made nonsense of the adult's harsh insistence on mark-making having to be some sort of picturing. Why should the paper have to have an 'on the wall' position? There are no necessary 'ups' or 'downs' on these marked rectangles of paper. Few of such marked papers would be intended to be a picture as we know it. Our limited view requires something as upon a screen or as seen through a window; we do not expect the 'drawing' to be a survivor of imaginative play. We do not even explore the wonderful possibilities of the process, we simply expect a rigid 'view' to be pinned upon the wall. One little boy I observed drew a set of lines upon a sheet, then bent it in part over the edge of a table, holding a pencil against that lowered part of the paper. He then moved the paper end and the pencil up to a horizontal position upon the table with much "brumm brumm" mechanical verbalisation. "This," he said, "is a crane lifting up a giant pencil." So it is that the paper can be folded and marked to play a temporary role. When it comes to mark making, the infant is not as limited as we are.

In trying to copy a face in profile when only one eye and one ear is visible, the child just has to draw two eyes and two ears, because a face has two eyes and two ears! The face, even in profile, is 'face as a subject', not 'face as an object' to the child. The profiled face clearly is 'face' and the child does not copy but represents the subject. Thus the visual misunderstanding is simply the child being 'subjective'. The sophisticated good copy of a profile is object-representation, the 'objective'. This is better demonstrated when a child draws a path with no perspective. The lines never meet and in a child's drawn representation look like a pillar to the adult beholder. When the path lines are drawn in perspective they may eventually meet on the horizon but the infantile and subjective drawing indicates that the lines do not meet. The objective drawing shows the lines meeting. So it is that we bring an 'objective' perception to a 'subjective' expression! How we muddle ourselves when we look at an infant drawing.

I could give other examples. Usually perspectival issues are included, for example, in perspective a circle on a plane is drawn as an oval. How can a circle be oval?

An 'objective' adult may even intrude into the child's feelings which are essentially subjective and when, for example, copying letters he or she may ignore adult 'up' and 'down' concepts and conventions, which easily results in reversals and even mirroring effects. This can frustrate teachers. It is easier for a child to write upside down than it is for most adults. A child will draw a complete figure 'upside down' for us. If we do not see the process we simply place the picture 'right way up' for us.

Interestingly we agreed, the Danish students and I, that it was quite amazing to realise that children in mark play might be given from their marking activity a fairly permanent reminder of their active existence; the experience of the play of their hands across the paper affording possible consideration of their four senses (touching, seeing, hearing, smelling and perhaps additionally tasking!) and four dimensions (point, line-plane, space and time). All this before the adult places the 'picture' upon the wall and tries to view it within 'limiting objectivity', seeing it as something of a window with a definite up and down.

Here is an example from my filming which shows how very special infant art is and how we can mislead ourselves in seeing 'picturing'.

Josh, at two years and ten months, describes to us how his artwork, which appears to be a crude figurative face-like drawing, is in fact a shop. He points out the counter (we had thought it was the mouth!) from which, in mime, he distributes imaginary biscuits and sweets. Next, on another sheet he produces, with a felt pen, 'spotting'. Each spot, he says, is something different. One is "a bird", another "Batman" and another is "a monster"! The other spots are even more wonderful; one is "a fast boom boom – it's up!" and there is even a (sung) "ob-dig-bed-ob!"

Josh, on the same occasion when asked to draw a face, obliges with a sweeping loop and marks it inside with three marks: a face. This seems easy but not so exciting for him and clearly less expressive than the other 'scribbles'.

I have in my investigations seen that children continue to re-create a favourite abstract shape while, within the same period, producing infantile 'figures' – often referred to by adults as 'stick men', 'potato men' or 'tadpole men'. Given a chance, children still continue to develop their (not so much loved by grown-ups) exploratory scribbles and patterns like Josh. So it does appear that the infant within art activity does not follow the supposed linear development but ranges widely to and fro, backwards and forwards, with his or her broad repertoire.

As I have seen in art therapy, clients young and old often use mysterious shapes and patterns (those we like to call 'abstract'). These may or may not connect with their mysterious infantile patternings (I think that it is very likely that they often do) but certainly contain expression. Usually the artist is able to give us clues as to what the expression is about. My unpublished research has helped me and many of my colleagues to develop a very respectful attitude to 'infantile non-representational configurations' created by young minds.

All in all we must proceed with great caution when we bring our rigid perception to the flexible world of infantile marking and drawing.

In my work in psychiatry I have to consider my limitations when I observe a little child making marks. It is fortunate for me that usually the child will help me to understand. I remind myself continually not to project something from me into their apparently ambiguous configurations, although in other publications about child art and art therapy it can often be seen that the author has not been able to resist this temptation!

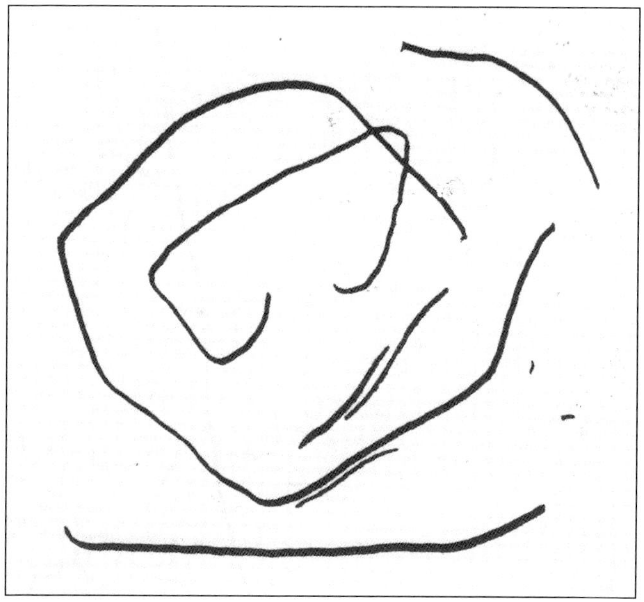

Not *a face. Josh's "shop"*

Chapter 14

Paul and the Wolf

A boy's complexity of communication

Many children I have worked with have briefly in their fantasies imagined themselves as a creature such as a monkey or a lion, but I have never met anyone like Paul who without hesitation would tell stories about friends and acquaintances as if they were all animals. When he repeated his tales he would always remember the animal that he had chosen to represent the person.

Nine-year-old Paul himself was, he said, 'the Cuttlefish', his close friend was 'Gorilla', a boy who sat near to him in class 'Monkey' and a girl was 'Pig'. I was also introduced to 'Seal', 'Crab', 'Giraffe' and 'Rabbit'. Interestingly, I was not to be an animal to Paul. First of all I appeared in his stories as 'The Man' but I eventually became 'Trevor' amongst the creatures. When this occurred I was delighted and felt that, because communication between myself and Paul was in the early days of our work together so difficult to establish, a change had occurred somewhere along the way. I had, it seemed, passed some sort of test and Paul was now allowing me into his stories as a friend and an observer but never a participator. Although I met with the other pupils in this residential school for children with emotional and behavioural difficulties, he seemed to be quite unique in this creativity.

Music

In retrospect, it seems that my early use of singing to a guitar to gain Paul's interest gained my access to his world. All the children in the school, whatever their problem, loved music and liked me bringing a guitar to the sessions, something I have very rarely felt the need to do.

Paul ignored my attempts to encourage him to pick up art materials. He would turn away and suck his thumb and hum a little. It was the tuneful humming that made me decide to bring the guitar along. Unthinkingly I started to play and sing 'Old MacDonald Had A Farm', which Paul stutteringly joined in with and introduced (not an ideal farm animal perhaps) the Giraffe, which at the end of the song he explained was his teacher. At that point no further comment about his 'animal friends' was made; that was to come later in our sessions when he began to draw.

'Doggy In The Window' was our next song; it became a duet. Here was a different side to the normally quiet and withdrawn Paul. 'Horsey, Horsey Don't You Stop' was followed by 'Three Little Fishes'. Thankfully I had an appropriate repertoire due entirely to my sing-alongs with my own young sons and daughter.

File Notes

It was after this early session, when I felt that I had now made a connection with Paul, that I decided to read his notes in the school's filing room, which was available to me at any time. I had already discovered that, because notes and letters come from well-meaning adults and often from a number of professionals, they did not describe the child's world in the way that the child might if he or she were able to supply their own notes! This might seem a minor point but it is, in my view, a significant one. After reading notes and referral letters, the therapist, doctor, social worker or whoever might take on a supposition as a fact. As far as possible, and if possible, with care and patience the adult may learn from the child a clue to what the problem really is.

In some cases, as we have seen earlier in the book, the encouraged expressiveness of the young person can explain the problem and can even fully or in part heal the child. One of many instances of misinformation comes to mind: a child that I had met had been described in the referral letter as severely emotionally disturbed by his grandmother's death, which had been followed by the news that his father was to have surgery. Art therapy sessions followed without questioning but from pictures, descriptions and eventually following very personal metaphoric stories, the truth emerged. First, he was "okay about Gran because she's with the angels and her nice friends". Secondly, "Daddy will be fine – he's tough". (Some worries there however, I thought) but thirdly he was so worried, he said, about Mummy and her new baby, because Mummy had been poorly and then baby sister had become poorly. Then Mummy was poorly again. Will they constantly take turns in being poorly? Will mummy be able to turn to her son with her love again? A distracted mum. A confused boy with a story of concern and perhaps some jealousy. A story which he could not share with the family. The concerns were revealed, with the boy's permission, to the mother and all was well. The child was reassured. But there was no great problem about Grandmother and Father dominating the boy's emotions and any focus on that, from the G.P.'s innocent letter, would have been something of a wild goose chase!

Like all the thirty pupils at this small residential school, Paul had a thick file with his history clearly defined. His disability was very much a mixture; difficult birth, delayed developmental milestones, too disruptive to continue with nursery/playgroup, unable to focus in school. Within all this was Paul's specific difficulty in communicating, often ranging from withdrawn silent periods to shouting and screaming outbursts with fewer and fewer periods lately between these extremes. In calm periods however, he learned in the classroom and was able to demonstrate how well he learned. Generally, then, Paul was seen as a child with 'emotional and learning difficulties'. The latest notes in the file suggested that over the last few months his behaviour had deteriorated, with a very noticeable increase in the number of angry outbursts. Because he was not doing so well he was referred to me, the 'visiting art therapist', with the hope that he might 'have the opportunity to give vent to his anger through art'. This note seemed a little alarming but this was, I suppose one way to perceive art therapy. Personally I had hoped that he would in some way express his anger symbolically and even talk about it without 'giving vent'!

I read on. There were well-founded theories regarding unprovable but likely brain damage ('neurological dysfunction'), resulting from difficulties before and during birth, being the root of many of Paul's problems. Notes from social workers on Paul at the age of nine described a nearly destitute family situation with a brother of four and an out-of-work father quite severely affected by tuberculosis. Apparently every family member took medication as a 'preventative' because of the father's illness. Paul's mother had mental health problems – there was a mysterious reference to her 'past traumatic experiences'. There were two sons from her first marriage, who were in care. One of these, Harry, (then fourteen years of age) had lately on two or three occasions during school holiday periods, returned to stay with his mother. There was a theory that he seemed jealous of his mother's attentions to Paul when they were all together and he could be aggressive to Paul.

As usual with such information, I turned to thoughts on the ongoing mysteries of 'Nature or Nurture'. Clearly Paul was, even as a small baby, disadvantaged by damage and trauma; this was sadly his 'nature'. But the 'nurture' (or lack of good nurturing) in the world he was born into was likely to have disabled him more. How could I help Paul? Frankly I was not sure that I could but I did remember advice given to me by a headteacher who had very special experience and knowledge of autistic children. She described her special pupils as having a 'core' problem from birth, but the attention they did or did not receive and their perceptions further complicated their condition as the years passed by. In time difficult nurture could severely exaggerate difficult nature. The headteacher was very much in favour of art therapy, because, she said, of its non-presumptuousness and the joy that she saw it bring to the children in her care. There had been in her life's work great improvements seen, she said, when art therapists worked with her pupils. This was to me a sort of 'layers of the onion' situation. Art therapy was not 'curing' the core problem, such as autism or learning difficulties, but removed some of those acquired outer negative layers.

Making Contact

So it was that I decided that my somewhat limited sessions (six) with Paul might be helpful. As it happened it was actually what Paul came to share with me and the change that followed because of that sharing that was the surprising and very positive outcome of my work. A bonus to the practical changes that were eventually made might be that Paul would feel a relief from his important sharings in art therapy and self-realisation of a developing ability to share more and more; improved communication and less frustration.

My first visit to Paul's residential school was merely to look around and to meet up with him. He was pointed out to me by a member of the care staff. Like most of the children Paul was enjoying his playtime by running about. He was quite small for his age, with dark scruffy hair and a wet nose. I stood at the edge of the crowd of children and watched a tall girl trying to hold him. He laughingly spun away, shouting, "Run! Run! Run!" On his next circuit Paul could not avoid the girl, who spat upon him. He did not seem to care but continued intent on his movements and not relating to anyone, not even a friendly member of staff who was on duty in the playground.

Surprisingly, I quickly caught his eye, I suppose because I was a new face in school. He moved towards me and grunted a few times. Eye contact was good as he said, quite clearly, "Who are you?" and gently held my arm. Now face to face, he shouted excitedly, "Look at me! Look at me!" Of course I was already looking at him. Next he made odd flicking tongue protrudings and pointed to his tongue repeatedly with his right forefinger. This was a ritual which I would see often repeated, sometimes with the pointing hand brought near to his tongue as he briefly licked his hand and fingers. Generally however, Paul presented himself to me in a friendly way but although I was trying, I could not strike up a conversation.

Just when I thought nothing else would happen there in the playground I heard a bell ringing; playtime was over, time for lessons. But as if the bell brought some magic, Paul began talking and gesturing in a very normal way, pointing to me and chatting. Ignoring the bell for a moment or two, I responded to his sensible enquiries: "Why are you here?" "What is your name?" "Will you come here lots of times?" and so on. Suddenly Paul seemed very able and as he eventually sped off to enter the school building I thought how good it would be to work with him.

The Sessions

Well it was good, and challenging, to work with Paul. He found it difficult to focus and was not very happy with the idea of art at first but he came to enjoy making drawings and stories to go with them. Perhaps my guitar and our songs were the breakthrough.

One difficulty in the sessions was the distraction of Paul's odd and unpredictable chantings, for example, "La la loo look look!" and "Dobby Obby Obby", fidgetings and hand lickings, which were, I realised, comforting rituals that he had learnt over the years. As time went on he resorted less to these rituals in the art room but sadly he remained as usual oddly-behaved about the school and dormitories.

Paul had an odd way of partly humming and partly singing. Although there were inexplicable phrases such as "Say macaroni", "Run and run and run" and "The Milky Bar", Paul's singing made melodic sense. I began to see that here was an intelligence that was masked by his odd behaviours and confused communication.

This was further demonstrated when Paul tired of our music-play and picked a book from a shelf. He showed me the pictures. I pointed out a colourful illustration saying, "Look – there's an octopus." Paul reprimanded me with a critical gaze, "It is not an octopus! This is a squid." Of course he was right. How clearly he had corrected me. Then, in a rather strange way he again recited a list of his animal friends, including himself, the "Cuttlefish", and a new addition, "The Man". After this he scribbled a pattern which had no meaning to me with some coloured pastels and the pen, ignoring the guitar now lying on the table. He was quiet again as the session came to an end.

Next time, although the guitar was in the room, Paul appeared not to notice and actually asked for his 'pictures'. I had them ready and he sat quietly at the table, choosing to use my pen to work with, rather than crayons and paint. He tired a little so I gathered the papers together and tried to get Paul to make a sort of picture book. He smiled and asked me to draw his animals. I did my best but from there on he scribbled and drew without asking me to contribute. Much of his drawing was not representational, at least not to me, usually a slowly meandering line sometimes taking on a shape. Although Paul was nine, his pictures at times seemed to be similar to a four-year-old's. Some odd loops were named by him, now the very much concentrating artist, as "Terry's pet", "Black widow spider shark", "Octopus shark with its mother", "A Verler with one eye", "Pond pet [within an added round enclosure] no eyes underwater", "The enormous bee stinger", and "Paul's pet – no eyes". "The Man" was mentioned but not drawn.

Over the following sessions markings were named and there were some special sharings such as The Man who, Paul laughingly revealed, was "You, Trevor!" He was quick to remind me to note what he was saying about it all.

Without this note-taking – and I felt good that Paul encouraged me to be his amanuensis – I believe that the important finale of Paul's story might never have been reached. In what follows I will attempt to recount the ongoing story, beginning with the re-introduction of the creatures that Paul had spoken of earlier, with a few added characters. After this, Paul moved on from Giraffe, Pig and company to focus on 'Wolf' and, surprisingly, 'Boy'. The latter I was sure was Paul.

The Story

So the story begins with a collection of animal friends. Next, two creatures with "a Mummy" emerge. Shark and Octopus are mentioned as marks are made, which Paul calls "Pebbles". Later I am told, without any illustration, that two sharks had killed the "Arm-Chopper Sharks" and "Jaws". I presumed that Paul had seen the movie Jaws. Apparently the two killer sharks next decide to fight each other.

Then I hear once more of the Giraffe, Octopus, Squid, Gorilla and Cuttlefish (Paul). Again no drawings, just the story. I am told that they all fight together but there seems to be no interesting outcome. Paul distracts himself and does lots of rather violent scribbles which contain, I think, half-a-dozen figures, letter forms (no words discernable) and creatures. Then, to Paul's great satisfaction, he creates a line on paper and when he stops to look at it (I see no figuration) he proudly tells me, "This is the enormous bee-stinger with big wings – they have a sharp knife."

The next moment, perhaps the most important moment in the therapy, Paul put my pen down and looking into the distance, spoke particularly clearly and quietly in a thoughtful way: "I let the Wolf stay with me because it was my friend. I let the Brown-Pig with the funny hair in. The Wolf went to sleep with me." Paul spoke so very seriously. I was puzzled and I thought of little pigs, the wolf, Red Riding Hood and the many wolf and fox stories that I had read over the years to my own children.

In a later session, when a description of real events were, I felt, becoming clarified, Paul asked me in a kind of sad way whether we could make many more 'drawing stories', words I am sure I had not used. Paul was teaching me that in therapy some stories cannot be just spoken but have to take on, in a way, something of a form of a novel with a necessary kind of beginning, middle and ending. There also had, it seemed, to be a special pace to these metaphorical, or semi-metaphorical expressions.

I had got into a habit of back-tracking the story, reading through our previous notes at the beginning of each session. On this occasion when I reached the part about the Wolf and the Pig, Paul exclaimed, "I punched the Wolf!" Rightly or wrongly my instant response was, "I thought that the Wolf was a friend. Why was he punched?"
"He just had to be punched," Paul replied, now looking into the distance with pen poised over his blank paper. Time passed. I broke the silence eventually and asked him if he would like to draw the Wolf. Without hesitation, Paul drew a simple primitive face followed by a busy dark scribbling beneath it. Very seriously, as he briefly placed the pen upon the table, he put his finger onto the drawn face and looked me directly in the eye. "The Wolf!" he dramatically declared. Picking up the pen again he carefully drew a rectangle which he said was "Paul's bed". (Not "a bed", nor "my bed".) I thought that it might be more uncomfortable to talk about "me" and "mine" than to use his own name.

Next came a circle with a simple figure without arms inside it. Pointing again to the figure he said, "He's sad!" Paul then drew a long line from his figure to the Wolf-face. "He's punched the Wolf!" he exclaimed with delight. This seemed to end the story but of course I was hoping for more. There was a surprise. After a minute or two, looking away from the drawing, Paul said, "The Wolf got punched because he bit me and Marie."

This was rather confusing. I was glad that I had not asked questions. Information was flowing from this little fellow and its expression, I felt, should give him some relief. The mystery was that this description, real or imagined, now included Marie.

Later I checked my notes and although I had heard of

Pig, Paul had not said that this was Marie. Perhaps Paul's experience of the Wolf reminded him of the vulnerability of Marie, a school companion he might be close to.

Since working with Paul I have come to understand that art therapy is not a jumbled jigsaw puzzle with all the pieces waiting to be slotted neatly into place. We have to adjust to the fact that some pieces do not fit and that others may be lost.

I heard nothing more of Marie but the story continued in a very clear and distressing way. Paul turned away from the drawing and, it seemed, ignored me, simply staring into the distance. With an unusually clear voice he announced, "The Wolf pulled the boy's trousers and pants down. The boy punched him on the nose. He smacked my bum. Paul ran away with no clothes." I was very surprised. All was quiet and now Paul was looking at me in a very calm way. I did not know what to say but I blurted out, "Then what?" He smiled and said, "Then Paul went to tell Trevor what happened!" I was moved by this.

Of course, because of his difficulties, especially his problems with communication, Paul might not have been able to tell his story. Even without disability we know that people treated badly, especially children, often irrationally blame themselves and find it difficult to tell their story. Paul's imagination, his animal friends and enemies, my pen, my guitar and, I suppose, his trust in me, were now allowing facts to emerge from his complex metaphors.

After a pause he added, "The boy was laughing," and Paul did laugh after making this statement. He continued laughing for a while but it was very strained and theatrical, disturbing. Then Paul took up the pen and started to draw an oval with a line beside it which, like the arm drawn on paper earlier, meandered to and fro for some length. This line next took on a curve and with increasing speed spiralled darkly into the centre as Paul concentrated. I saw and felt sadness. A dark spiral has been drawn in front of me by a number of depressive people over the years. It is a hole, even a darkness, which is so difficult to get out of. Was this an expression of how Paul, not really a laughing boy, felt? Of course, his fluctuating function of mental ability, between four and nine years, precluded the possibility that the words 'distressed', 'depressed' or 'melancholy' could be available to him for expression.

So what of the spiral and my reaction? I managed to say nothing as Paul looked at it and commented, "I went down the hole! It really was a hole. I went down the rude hole with no clothes on." Paul pointed to the centre of his spiral and commented strangely, "The hole says... 'Be rude outside... like my brother... Really?'" Silence followed. There was no more drawing. Was Paul's depressive feeling suggesting that he should be just like his brother? Knowing that this was our penultimate session and with an idea that Paul might be, or had been, sexually abused, I risked direct questioning to gain helpful information.

"What happens to the Wolf?" I prompted. "I chuck him out. Of the window and punch him." Paul shrugged his shoulders and smiled. I felt like he was saying something like, "That's it! The story is over." Then loudly he proclaimed, "Everyone is chucked out of the window!"

To my surprise Paul stood up and tidied the table top. He was clearly finished and in fact our time was up. We said our goodbyes and as I watched the boy leave, it seemed that he was indicating that there was nothing more to tell.

In our last session, however, I was quite surprised to discover that the story was not complete. Somehow at this beginning I was not picking up the papers and re-reading Paul's tale back to him. I did not, as it happened, need to. He walked into the room, confidently said, "Hello, Trevor," sat down and immediately started to draw. A crude and undetailed figure with eight limbs appeared.

In a calm and clear way that we could not have seen in earlier sessions, where he presented as very much a special needs and difficult pupil, he began to talk me through the primitive picture before I could question him: "Paul comes out of the hole!... And... out of the window. No clothes on!" He waited for me to respond. I did: "Tell me about this, please." I pointed to the eight-limbed shape. Paul seemed happy to answer, "Paul is touching. He is the Octopus-Spider!" Not so very different from his earlier form of Cuttlefish, I thought. The touching element seemed important.

Turning to a fresh piece of paper Paul produced another spiral, this time scribbling vigorously in its centre. In a theatrical way and with a surprisingly deep voice, he slowly pronounced, "Down the Dark Hole." He seemed to be saying that because of the Wolf, he was still down the dark hole. The Wolf had entered the story as a friend and I remembered that in fairy tales during the first meeting or two with the wolf, friendliness is shown, for instance the enquiring wolf in the woodland meeting with Red Riding Hood. Happily I was not lost in such distractions because Paul began another drawing with another spiral, this time not condensing but taking on shapes, all of which were quite meaningless to me.

Paul stopped and pointed to one of the shapes, saying, "The Wolf with no eyes." Another little shape he called, "Paul" and again the exclamation, "Wolf pulled trousers and pants down! Wolf pulled trousers and pants down!" He paused and then continued in a sad way, "I never cried. He went to bed with me. He took my clothes off."

Paul turned away from the table and looked at me for the first and only time with tearful eyes. "The Wolf is so bad!" he sobbed. I could not help asking, "Who is the Wolf?" Should I have known better? Only because this was our last session I needed to risk bringing the tale out of metaphor. If I could discover who the Wolf was I could see to it that Paul would be protected. Of course Paul replied, "The Wolf is the Wolf." I was not really surprised at this.

Carefully, taking his time, Paul took another piece of paper and stared at its blankness for a time before drawing. He made yet another spiral, this time in the corner and quite small, "Brother Harry says 'Poo! Poo!'" I remembered that I had heard of brother Harry earlier when The Hole advised Paul to be rude outside like his brother. Harry, I knew from Paul's file, was the older brother who attended another residential special school but in the past few months had spent periods at home, possibly sharing a bedroom with Paul.
A new piece of paper and another spiral, more dense this time, and a mark which could have been a crude stick man figure inside. Paul surveyed his drawing as he spoke. I found it difficult to believe I was hearing what was spoken with such determined and unhurried clarity. Paul said as he again looked me in the eye, "That's me. I'm trapped!"

He then took another piece of paper and scribbled a rough circle, not so much a spiral and seemed to brighten up. "Brother has the wheel," he said and then made some little separate looping lines. "Funny Hats!" then a pause, then he laughed. "Poo! Poo!" I could make no sense of this and felt a little frustrated as I heard the children moving out of the classroom next door and into the playground. This was our last session, our last moments and there was to be no resolution to please me, the therapist. Paul clearly wanted to go to play. He said a smiling, "Bye, Trevor," and walked out of the room to play with his friends.

Before the end of playtime I went to Paul to say goodbye and wish him well. I felt bad that he had apparently said that he was "trapped" but I could tell Paul's school of the likelihood of sexual abuse by his brother – I was now convinced of this. They would then ensure that he would be protected. I hoped also that in the near future he would become less distressed and his more recent angry behaviours (never seen in our sessions) would diminish.

Reporting on my Findings

Although I was unable to attend a multi-disciplinary meeting regarding the concerns I had expressed to the headteacher on my last day, I did present a full report. No-one had suspected that Paul might be suffering from abuse at home. The consultant psychiatrist was fully convinced, however, as was the social worker attached to the school. I was very pleased, of course, that my report had been taken seriously despite notes of 'sing-alongs' with the art therapist and tales of Giraffe, Cuttlefish and Wolf.

Later, contacts from the school informed me that Paul's brother had made some form of confession to the police but prosecution seemed unlikely. Social Services had ensured that Paul would be safe from now on and his name was placed on the Child Protection Register.

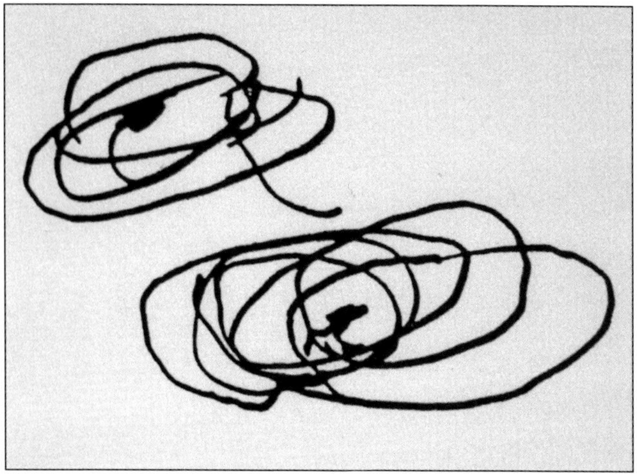

Outcomes

The outcome of this art therapy was helpful because important information was gathered which helped the boy. In the following few months I did have a problem because, I think, at the back of my mind at this time I thought that my work should really be 'detective work'. Luckily I came to realise that this was wrong. I believe that an art therapist may, perhaps be put briefly in the role of detective when the client is struggling to ask for help. Unfortunately, much if not all of the therapeutic possibilities will vanish if the therapist is in that narrow role of information seeker. Our job is to provide, without presumption, a welcoming empty space for the client to fill with whatever they desire to fill it with.

I learned something extra from my time with Paul. The member of the school's care staff who had special responsibility for Paul seemed rather angry with me when I told her of my findings. This I could not understand because I was so very careful with my words when I spoke to her. I concluded that there was something about my demeanour that she disliked. A year or so later I came to understand what was behind the anger. My good friend, the child psychiatrist Dr Margaret Wright, who found me my first position in NHS work and encouraged me greatly, explained this to me when two mothers seemed to dislike me while I was working in her clinic. The explanation made sense because I clearly had an expectation that parents would certainly appreciate my work.

Dr Wright asked me a good question, along the lines of, "How would you feel if someone so very close to you shared so little with you and then went off into an art room with a strange man and expressed feelings from the depths of their soul? Would you be put out?" Yes, it is very likely that I would.

Brave Therapists

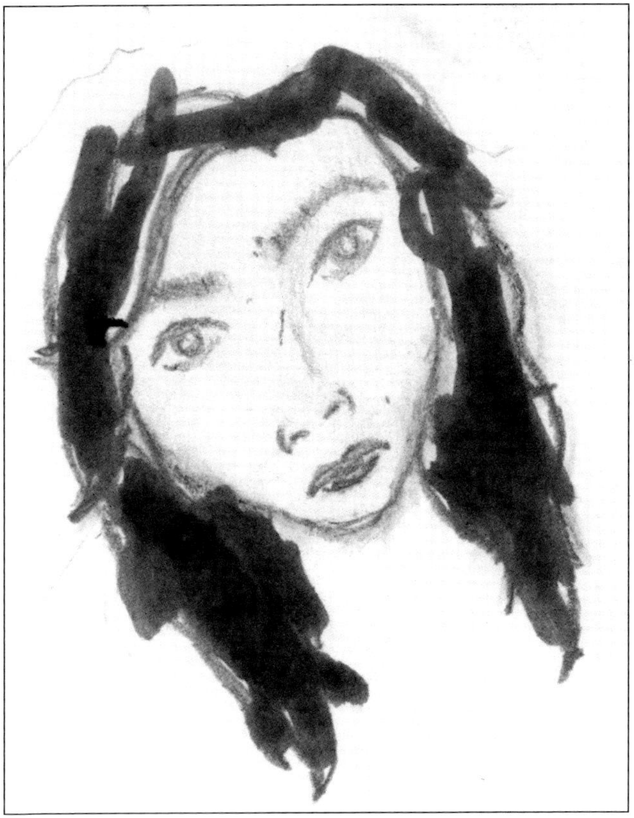

I was once asked by an art therapist that I was training, "Is there one thing that is necessary to be a therapist?" Immediately, almost without consideration, I replied to this question that I had not heard before, "You have to be brave."

Looking back this was, I am very sure, the best simple answer. We have to believe in our work, believe in ourselves (with the realisation that we will not always be correct or perfect), be brave in what we do and not expect to fully understand what is actually happening. We try to help. A positive outcome is what matters, not the gathering of 'interesting' material, not to be seduced by the images but always to keep in mind that we work as people doing our best to help through encouragement.

I was very impressed years ago by the pioneer American art therapist Edith Kramer who, like myself and others, was lecturing at a seminar in Denmark. Edith joined speakers at a question session at the end of the weekend and at one point we were all asked about how we worked. Some described aspects of neurological functions, others complex theories and some talked of what their university training brought to their work. Edith simply said, "I try to help children."
As for myself, I hope I have been, at least for much of my time working with young people, a 'friendly enabler' and within that I've had to be brave enough to follow what I feel, rather than theoretical structures.

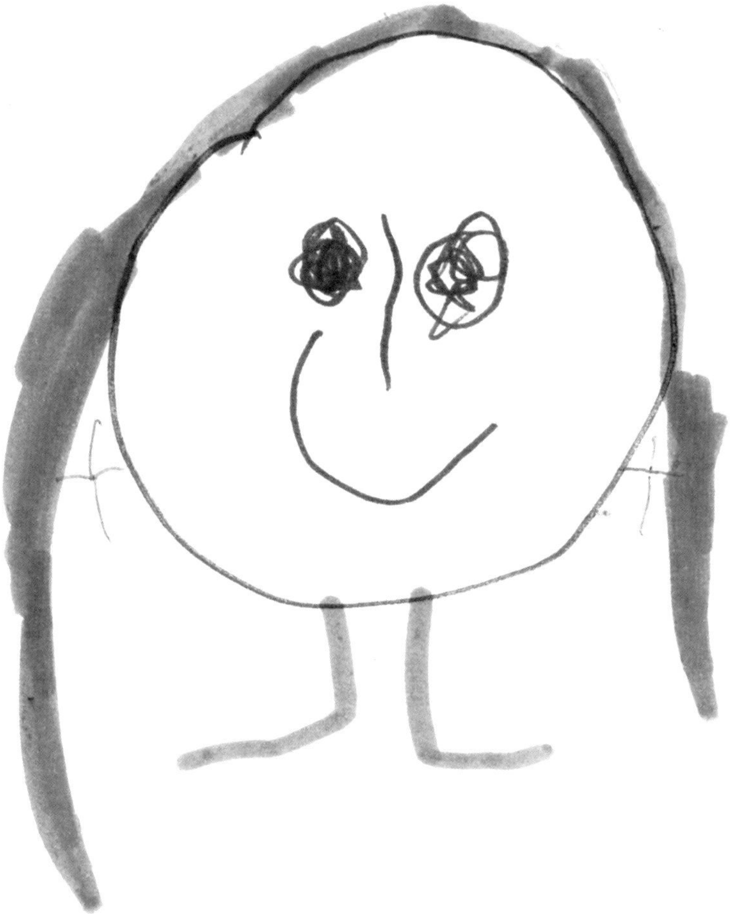